BOSH!
HEALTHY VEGAN

BOSH!
HEALTHY VEGAN

HENRY FIRTH & IAN THEASBY

WM
WILLIAM MORROW
An Imprint of HarperCollins*Publishers*

HarperCollins books may be purchased for educational, business, or sales promotional use. For information, please email the Special Markets Department at SPsales@harpercollins.com.

Originally published in Great Britain in 2020 by HQ, an imprint of HarperCollins Publishers Ltd.

FIRST U.S. EDITION

Design & Art Direction: Hart Studio
Food photography: Lizzie Mayson
Portrait photography: Nicky Johnston
Food styling: Pip Spence
Prop styling: Louie Waller
Recipe Nutritional Consultant: Clare Gray
With thanks to Newington Green Fruit & Vegetables

Library of Congress Cataloging-in-Publication Data has been applied for.

ISBN 978-0-06-296993-4

20 21 22 23 24 LSC 10 9 8 7 6 5 4 3 2 1

CONTENTS

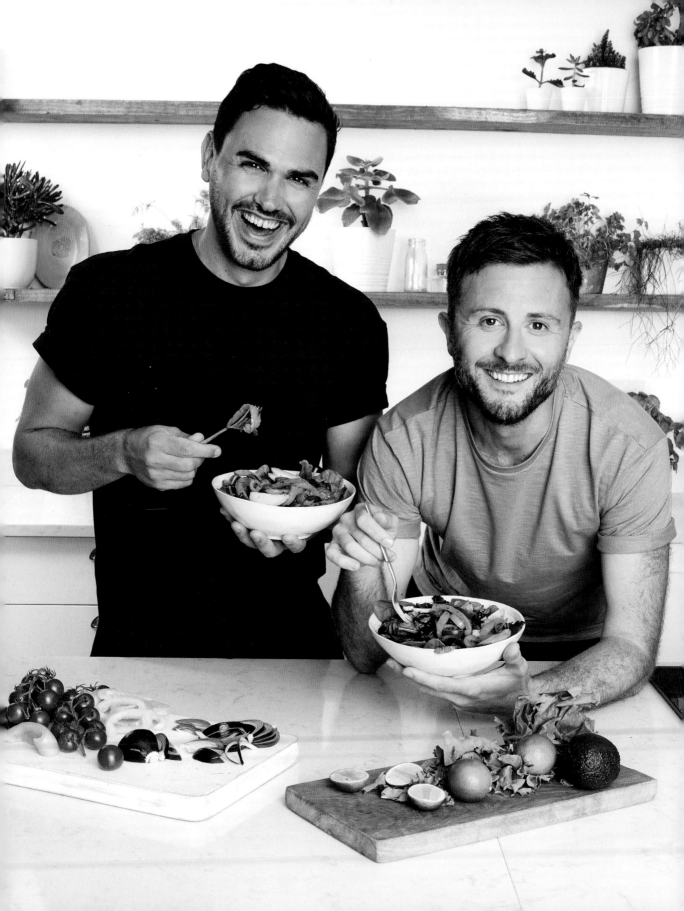

WELCOME

As BOSH!, it's our mission to help you get more plants on your plate, more taste in your food, and more joy out of your mealtimes. We want you to live a long, healthy, happy life. Our aim in this book is to share with you what we've learned about healthy eating and the power of plants.

Four years ago, we were slightly overweight meaties. We adopted a plant-based diet and found our lives changed for the better. The weight fell off, our sleep was better, and our energy levels improved. But a couple of years later, we had become indulgent eaters, often cooking and eating up to five meals a day as we tested recipes for our cookbooks. We had taken our focus off health and well-being and were eating too many white, processed carbs—classic vegan junk food! It was delicious, but our health had started to suffer.

So, we made some changes and started learning a new way of living. We learned how to balance fun food with fit food. We've done the hard work—and made the mistakes—so you don't have to. In this book we share with you over 80 healthy recipes, meal plans, and all the advice and guidance you need to be a happier, healthier, leaner you—whether it's every meal, or one meal at a time.

But this isn't a diet book. Quick diets and promises of instant transformation don't work in the long term. If they sound too good to be true, that's because they are. With the latest diet craze you may see short-term benefits, but these can often be at the expense of your future self.

Quick-fix diet plans can lead to an unhealthy relationship with food, encourage a negative self-image, and even permanently change your body's metabolism. More often than not, once the diet is over you'll go back to your old eating patterns anyway and any benefits will be reversed. We've all been there.

We are going to show you how eating plants can transform your well-being, for good. Making a small change to the way you eat, you can feel incredible and live healthier. And the best part? The food is delicious!

When we adopted this plant-based way of eating, we felt more energetic, slept better, trained better, laughed a lot more, and, hopefully, we will live longer, too!

This book is for everyone, whatever your dietary lifestyle. Whether you're a vegetarian, a vegan, a flexitarian, a pescatarian, a meat eater—this book is for you. We'll show you how to eat the rainbow, whether you're looking to lose fat, eat for fitness, or just be the healthiest you can be. It's about finding the balance that you feel comfortable with and incorporating plant-based eating into your life as much as you can.

If you're looking to lose fat, become leaner, or shape up, a plant-based diet is one of the best ways to do that. Eating the right plants will help you feel fuller for longer, which can help you start to shed fat (see page 54).

If you're looking to build muscle, you're in the right place. Colorful plants are packed with protein and a load of vital nutrients to help you get maximum gains and experience optimum recovery after exercise. We'll show you how plant-based nutrition can help fitness and muscle building (see page 57).

If you're just looking to be a healthier version of you, then this is for you. We want to help everyone reach their optimum health. These recipes will help your gut, blood, heart, and immune system function at their best.

Our recipes are delicious, easy, and offer the best in nutrition. They have been put together using the latest medical advice available for a plant-based diet, and according to UK government guidelines (the EatWell Plate) and other national food guidelines. And we've worked with a registered dietician to make sure that all our dishes are balanced, health-giving, and well portioned.

The recipes all follow the principles of eating the rainbow. Packed with colorful plants and their unique health-giving phytonutrients, they reflect a varied plant-based diet. The meals are also full of dietary fiber and high-quality carbs, proteins, and fats, and are low in salt, sugar, and saturated fat (saturated fat has links with increased cholesterol, heart disease, and stroke, so a diet that's low in this is great!).

They have all been nutritionally analyzed—you'll see labels beneath the recipes indicating whether they are a particularly good source of protein or fiber, or are low in fat or sugar, as well as the calories per serving.

We'll show you why eating plants is a great choice for your health. You'll learn how to eat plants the right way, while discovering delicious new recipes. We'll also give you some ideas for when you want to relax the rules a little, so you can enjoy life in balance. We all need a treat sometimes!

We'll help you get healthy in other areas of your life as well—sleep, exercise, routine, and lifestyle—so you feel more able to to start making positive, lasting changes.

We're going to show you how to eat and live healthily. You'll soon see just how good you can feel eating plants. Most important, this is still BOSH! food: hearty, comforting food that you want to eat—but with fewer calories, less sugar, and less fat.

We're going to share with you everything we've learned and help you find the best you. These changes could last a lifetime. And along the way we'll share some of the tastiest and most vibrant recipes we've ever created.

We're delighted you've decided to join us on our healthy vegan journey.

Henry and Ian x

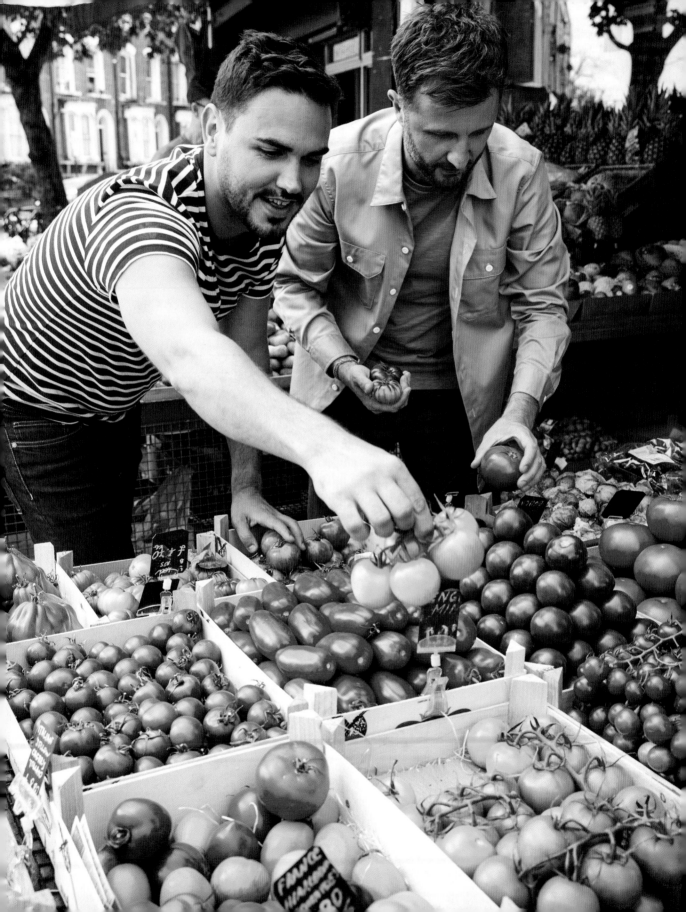

WHY EAT PLANTS?

In this book, you're going to discover delicious, moreish, comforting food that is good for your body, will nourish your soul, and will help you stay healthy. And moreover, everything is easy and you won't be spending ages in the kitchen.

You've probably heard that a plant-based diet is good for you. There's a reason many of the world's top athletes are adopting plant-based diets. It's the new buzzword in fitness. And it's being recommended increasingly by doctors as a lifestyle promoting long life, weight loss, and health.

We have found that it has loads of other benefits, too, like better sleep, improved recovery after exercising, and more consistent energy levels. It's better for the planet, too. We felt like we'd discovered a superpower when we first made the switch. We are now fitter, happier, and healthier than we've ever been.

PLANTS ARE GOOD FOR YOU

Your parents always told you to eat your greens, and they were right! Eating more plants is a sure-fire way to turbocharge your wellness: most plants are absolutely jam-packed with phytochemicals that have various positive benefits for the body, from offering anti-oxidizing properties, to providing vital vitamins and minerals (see pages 49–52), and supporting good gut health.

You may also find, as we did, that eating vegan, which is characterized by consuming more fiber and less of what are thought to be inflammatory foods, leaves you with better digestion and a healthier gut.

The easiest way to maximize nutrition on a plant-based diet is to remember to "eat the rainbow" (we talk more about this on pages 42–45). It's also best to avoid overprocessed foods as much as possible. Get a variety of colors, flavors, textures, and spices into your diet on a daily basis: aim for your plates of food to be beautifully colorful.

STILL EAT ALL YOUR FAVORITE FOODS

"Surely a vegan diet just means eating loads of salads and rabbit food? Lettuce and carrots, right?" We beg to differ! A good vegan diet, packed with health-giving properties and general planty goodness, can still be hearty and comforting.

We started BOSH! to show the world just how delicious plant-based food can be. We created our videos to prove that you can still have all your favorite foods, but without the meat and dairy. And with our new, healthy recipes, nothing's changed.

Incredible-looking burgers, luscious roast dinners, wonderful stews and curries, and even pizza can still be on the menu! And we're not talking about processed burgers or cauliflower-crust pizzas either. We're talking about proper hearty meals made as you like them, with just a few small tweaks to nudge the meal in a healthy direction.

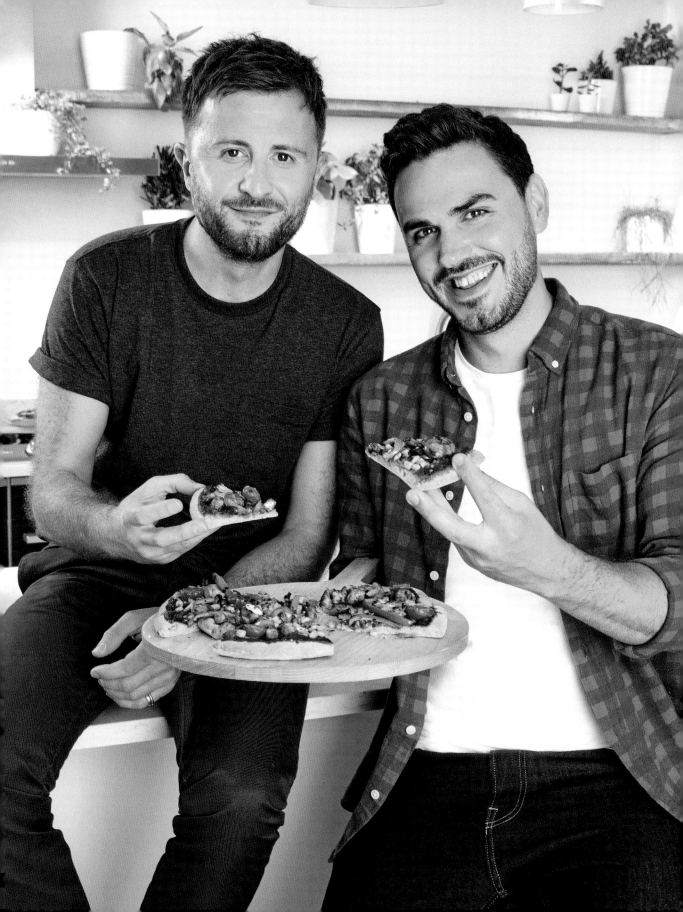

"Going vegan made me stronger than I've ever been . . .
I feel better than ever, I look and feel younger."

David Haye—British professional boxer

DITCH THE DIETS

We all know about those best-selling "healthy" or "fat-loss" cookbooks that contain meals packed with meats, fish, and cheese. Many are based on the same principles of the ketogenic or Atkins diets, which encourage your body to burn fat instead of glucose. These books and their exercise plans may result in weight loss in the short term, but chances are it will be short-lived. They may also be very high in fat and saturated fat.

And, if you aren't doing the exercise plans associated with these diets, then you may not even see the benefits. You could even end up putting on weight rather than losing it, due to the high caloric content of the food.

Crashing in and out of different diets with different approaches to weight loss, by eating less, or eating more fats and proteins, you could end up affecting your body's metabolism. Your body has an optimum balance, and it may adjust how it operates so it can remain there.

Unlike those diets, our approach to nutrition, healthy eating, and fitness is flexible. You don't have to be doing complicated aerobics routines every day. We're not saying you should avoid exercise—we are big advocates of it!—but our approach to eating works independently, with you moving and getting your body active in your own way. Perhaps a brisk walk to work or a bike ride to do your shopping is enough to get your heart beating faster. That's fine—you'll still feel the benefits from eating our meals. Or, if you are a regular gym bunny, then this book will work for you, too, and later on we'll show you how to tailor your meals to achieve your fitness goals (see page 57).

HEALTHY EATING IS FOR LIFE

This book will help you work through a few small changes to your lifestyle (and when we say small, we mean small) to steer yourself toward a happier, healthier you: one, two, three years from now. We hope this book will help you take control of your health, your body, your food, your energy levels, for once and for all.

By learning a few simple rules on how to nourish yourself on a plant-based diet, you can take the stress out of mealtimes for good. We certainly won't tell you what you should or shouldn't look like either. Loving your body as it is, right now, is more important than anything else.

THE PLANT SLANT

Until recently, concerns about nutrition put some people off a plant-based diet, and "vegan" was almost seen as a dirty word. Now, many doctors are moving toward recommending plant-based eating, and more health professionals are recommending plant-based–or as some people call it, "plant-slant"–diets to patients for promoting long life, fitness, weight loss, and better recovery from illness. Eating only plants–or a lot more plants–is now seen as the optimal way to eat. And it's better for the planet and all its inhabitants, too.

"I am a firm believer in eating a full plant-based, wholefood diet that can expand your life length and make you an all-around happier person."

Ariana Grande–pop star

VEGGIES ARE EASY TO COOK AND A GOOD VALUE

Vegetables are easy to cook and don't require long cooking times: you just need to learn how to make flavors work. We design our recipes with easy-to-find foods, so you can get most things from your local stores. And eating more plants can save you money, too. You don't need to worry about spending loads on expensive free-range meat. You just want fresh veg. And if you buy seasonal or discount items (plants stay good for longer), then your shopping can be even cheaper.

DO IT YOUR WAY

You may well not be vegan, but this book is still for you! The more plants you eat, the better. Maybe a totally plant-based diet is just not for you. Maybe later. Maybe never. This book is written for everyone, no matter how many plant-based meals you choose to eat each day or week.

"Not only does it help me on the court, but I feel like I'm doing the right thing for me. It definitely changed my whole life. It changed everything."

Serena Williams—world-class tennis player (on adopting a plant-based diet)

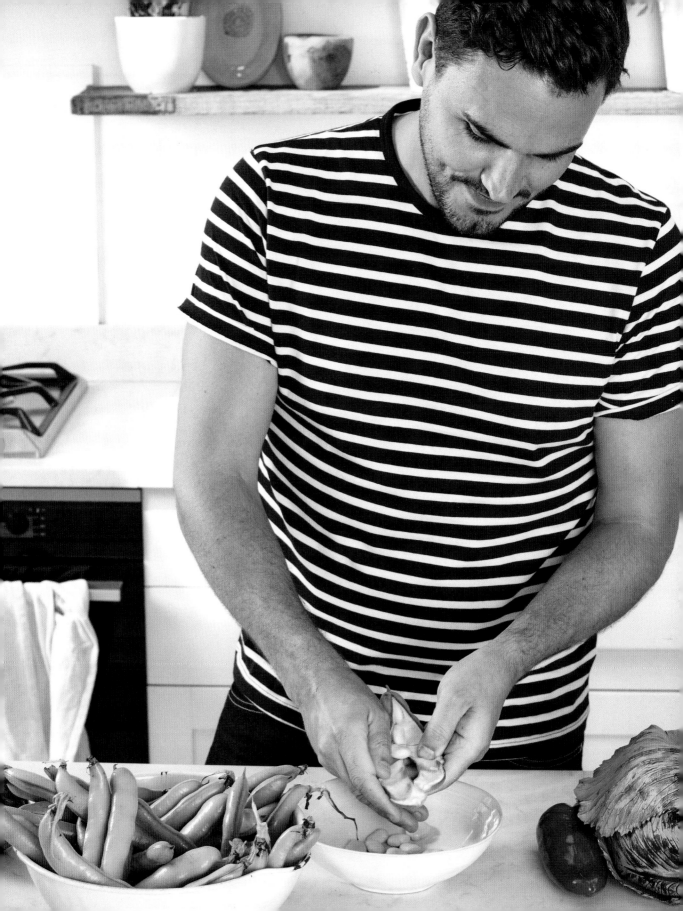

THE BOSH! STORY

The worst of times

In 2014, we were both in a bad place. Henry had just celebrated his thirtieth birthday. He woke up with "the fear," having forgotten everything about the night before, and tried to work out what had happened. Luckily, save for embarrassing himself, no real damage was done. But he was also a work-hard-play-hard kind of guy, and food and alcohol were taking a toll on his life. That was the wake-up call he needed.

Around a similar time, Ian was looking and feeling under the weather, and had been for a while. Carrying a little more weight than he wanted, and between jobs, he had lost all motivation. He denied that anything was wrong, but he was spending far too much time eating junk food and drinking, and not enough time looking after his body. And he was doing absolutely zero exercise. No running, no stretching, no cycling, no weights, not much walking. Nothing.

Both of us were making bad life choices. And these poor choices were making us unhealthy, unfit, and unhappy.

As January approached, Ian decided to give up alcohol as a personal challenge. He found it easier than he expected, so he decided to up the ante and give up meat, too. As part of that process, he started reading up on meat production, and watching veggie and vegan YouTube videos. And he decided to go vegan.

We lived together (and still do), and shortly after Ian decided to go vegan, we watched the film *Cowspiracy*. On discovering the environmental, health, and ethical impact of animal agriculture, Henry joined Ian and went vegan overnight, too.

Almost instantly, we both felt amazing. We lost a bit of weight. Our energy levels improved. We felt generally lighter, as our digestive systems were less strained. Our hair got thicker and we slept better. Henry's hay fever pretty much disappeared. We felt fitter and healthier than ever. Despite the fact that it was harder to find food (in 2014 there wasn't as much choice for vegans), we felt more satisfied and more fulfilled by our choices. The overall positivity of the vegan experience was intoxicating, and so we set up BOSH! to share our love of vegan food with the world.

The rest is vegan history. Within months we had millions of views of our videos. Within a year, billions.

However, there was a downside. While we were eating plant-based foods—which are, inherently, healthy—the sheer amount of food we were cooking and testing was causing us problems. We're incredibly proud of the food in our BOSH! books, but, put simply, we were eating too much! Particularly for Henry, those repeated tests to make the perfect lasagna or burger resulted in him piling on the pounds he had initially lost.

When you immerse yourself in the vegan world, you realize just how easy it is to make vegan versions of almost anything. This is a great thing, as it shows that vegan food doesn't need to be about abstinence. But, as any dietician or medium- to long-term vegan or vegetarian will tell you, it's easy to be an unhealthy vegan, or to just be eating the wrong things. After all, salad is vegan—but so are chips!

We found that cutting meat out of our diet was a great thing to do—it helped us eat less saturated fat, and encouraged us to bring more fiber and nutrients into our diet. A plant-based diet reduces your impact on the planet, and you know that what you eat doesn't contribute to poor animal welfare—but if you're not careful, you can easily end up low in key nutrients.

In addition to the overeating, our increasingly busy lives negatively affected our work-life balance. We had no time for exercise. Our hectic video production schedule meant we often didn't leave the house for days on end. When we did leave, we filled our faces with vegan burgers, vegan fish and chips, and brownies at vegan food events. Gradually we became unhealthier versions of our vegan selves, living on "junk food vegan" diets. At home, there were far too many take-out meals. Our meals were less "eat the rainbow" and more "50 shades of beige."

Time to change

At the start of 2018, we decided to get healthy.

It wasn't a big change. More a re-steering of the ship. We changed our course by a couple of degrees, watched our ship right itself, and found a completely new destination.

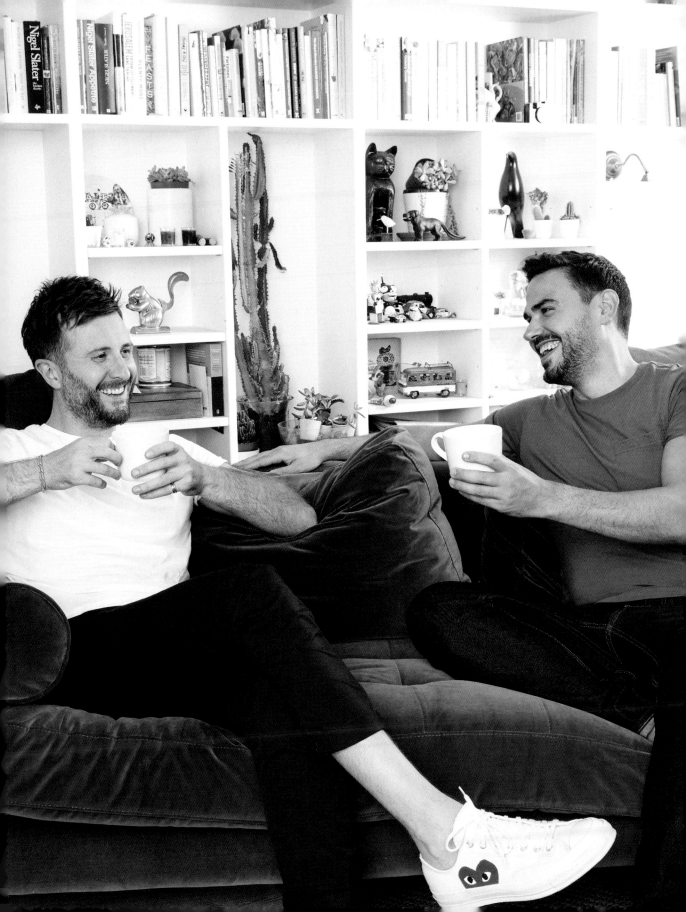

The best of times

We sought advice everywhere we could, reading dozens of books, watching videos and documentaries, following courses, and speaking to doctors and nutritionists. We sought out mentors. We started working with a dietician.

Our new way of eating and living focused on colorful plants, and getting the right balance of nutrients. This, as well as a small amount of careful supplementation, ensured we were getting exactly the right nutrition for our bodies.

Following our new meal plan felt great. We felt light and lean. We had successfully navigated ourselves to a place where we felt fantastic all week long, saved money, saved time on cooking, and were still able to eat the kind of meals we wanted (allowing ourselves to indulge in a vegan junk food session from time to time). We went to the gym regularly, and were better at getting up early. Our work has improved, our happiness has increased, and we are healthier than we have ever been.

This is the toolkit we wish we'd read when we were starting out on our vegan journey. We wish we'd known that by following just a few simple steps and basic rules we could ensure we achieved optimum nutrition from a plant-based diet.

A new you

Our goal is to help everyone in the world eat more plants. That's what we're about. It's what we've always been about. It's why we started BOSH! and why we've written our cookbooks.

We've updated our mission a little bit from where we started. As well as helping everyone eat more plants, we also want our recipes to inspire, entertain, and nourish, and we want to improve the health of the planet and all its inhabitants. If everyone adopted a plant-based diet, we could make a big contribution to reducing climate change.

That's why we're here, and it's why we created the recipes in this book. We're here to show the why and the how of living healthily on a plant-based diet.

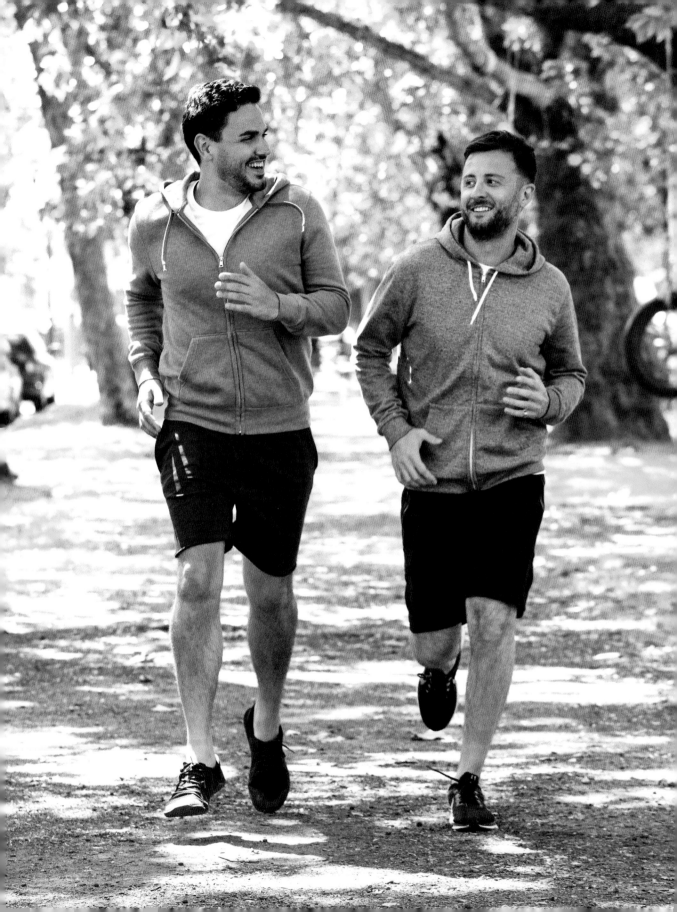

HOW TO LIVE WELL

A healthy lifestyle means different things to different people. But all of us will benefit from focusing on these six pillars:

- **sleep**

- **move**

- **relax**

- **love yourself**

- **love others**

- **live with purpose**

A long, healthy, happy life has all these bases covered. Don't compare yourself to others, but think about how well you feel when you follow the principles of each in your own life. We'd like to share with you some simple, meaningful changes you can make to live better.

SLEEP

Rest is crucial for your body. During sleep our body undergoes all sorts of essential activities. Doctors recommend we aim for between 7 and 9 hours per night–any less than this counts as sleep deprivation, which can have many negative health consequences. So getting good sleep is crucial.

One of the most positive changes we made was to improve our sleep. We used to get up early to hit the gym, even if it meant getting only 5 or 6 hours of sleep. We were spending our days sleep deprived, trying to catch up on the weekends.

But after learning about the impact sleep has on physical performance, we made time to sleep properly. Now we get 7 to 9 hours of good-quality sleep most nights and the difference to our lives has been incredible. Even if we hit the gym a bit less often, we see more benefits from the times we do go, and we eat more sensibly during the day, too, as we're less likely to need a quick energy boost.

Being sleep deprived is detrimental to your health. It can impair brain function, memory, and empathy. It negatively affects your mood and increases stress hormones. It is also more likely to cause us to make bad food choices, and since we're tired, we are more likely to skip exercise. Being tired impairs our body's ability to grow muscle and, conversely, makes us more likely to put on fat.

Of course, there are some jobs, such as doctors, nurses, chefs, or shift-workers, that require long and erratic working hours, or night shifts. This can make a regular sleep pattern an impossibility. In this case, getting the maximum sleep possible and the best-quality sleep you can (even including naps) will help you manage your rest time.

After a good night's sleep you'll reap many benefits, including more energy, higher concentration, and stronger learning ability. You'll be more likely to make good food choices and your body will be better at building muscle or burning fat. Your immune system and bodily repair systems will also improve. In his trailblazing book, *Why We Sleep*, Matthew Walker shows that you'll have better memory, increased life expectancy, lower stress levels, and more empathy. In addition to the food you eat, sleep is one of the biggest things we want to help you with.

How to sleep well

- **Create a bedtime ritual.** Go to bed and wake up at the same time every day—even on the weekends—if you can.

- **Keep your cell phone and TVs out of the bedroom,** using something else as your alarm clock. Ian likes to use a light alarm clock, and Henry likes to wake up to a motivational podcast to get him up and raring to go! We set up a charging point in the hallway for phones.

- **Reduce your caffeine intake.** We used to drink up to five cups a day—that's too many! Have your coffee in the morning, or at lunchtime, then it's out of your system by bedtime.

- **Reduce exposure to bad light at bedtime.** Looking at your phone or a computer screen late at night can make your body think it's morning, due to the bright blue light your devices emit. Try to turn off technology an hour or so before bed, or if you really can't do that, use an app that will dim the light of the screens. These are available on most cell phones, and you can download laptop applications to do the same thing.

- **Put yourself on a strict sleep routine.** Aim to get 8 hours of sleep a night, for a week, at the expense of all else (even exercise). See how amazing you feel. Then take it from there!

- **Aim to get your room as dark and quiet as possible at bedtime.** If your room isn't completely dark, try fitting blackout blinds or using a really comfortable eye mask. And ear plugs are great for helping keep sounds out—get the best ones you can.

- **Keep your room cool.** Around 65°F is a good temperature. If you find you are sweating, or tossing and turning, consider investing in a duvet with a lower thermal overall grade (TOG) rating.

- **Make your bed each day.** Your bed should be as inviting and as comfortable as possible. Invest in some quality fitted sheets and bedding that you love.

- **Embrace napping.** Napping is great, and it Is a skill that can be learned. A 20-minute daytime nap can do wonders to revive you; even a 5-minute nap can leave you feeling refreshed. Sofas, car seats, or even your desk at work can be great nap spots, where you can bring yourself back to alertness if you're a little low on sleep.

- **Get outside first thing in the morning and get 20 minutes of daylight** on your skin (not through glass, and not wearing sunglasses!). We find exercising in the morning (usually running or cycling) is a great way to do this, but see what works for you.

MOVE

There's a test called the sit-to-stand test, or sit-rising test, which is usually conducted on people over 50. It analyzes your overall mobility and balance, and is used to make predictions about how long you are likely to live based on your performance in the test. It involves going from standing to sitting on the floor, and then back up to standing without using your hands, arms, knees, or the side of your leg to support you. When Henry was 30, he realized he couldn't perform the simple movement in that test. It was at this point that he started regular exercise, including strength and mobility work.

Regular exercise is one of the top factors in ensuring a healthy body. Movement doesn't have to be overly taxing; even just walking briskly for 30 minutes throughout the day counts toward an active lifestyle. The UK government guidelines recommend adults aged 19 to 64 aim for 150 minutes of moderate exercise or 75 minutes of vigorous exercise each week, as well as strength exercises on two or more days a week. So, whether you're walking, running, stretching, or lifting, regular movement is crucial.

As the saying goes, "use it or lose it."

Most able-bodied toddlers can perform an excellent squat; humans are born with great mobility. Over time, in the West, we lose that ability—squatting just isn't something we do on a regular basis, compared to places like India and Southeast Asia, where squatting to sit is common, and you'll find most people can still perform a perfect squat. If you're not making full use of a range of motion, it will gradually stop being available to you.

The same applies to our muscles. Your body is an efficient machine, and if you're not using muscles, they will start to deteriorate. These changes are not immediately noticeable, but before you know it you can get a sprain from performing a simple task. Your muscles need to be adequately maintained across their whole range of movement, otherwise even a small movement outside of their norm can end up causing damage.

In addition to loss of mobility and strength, overly tight and inflexible muscles can cause damage elsewhere in your body, as you may be holding yourself awkwardly to compensate. Back pain is often actually caused by tightness in the legs and glutes, and the longer tightness is left unchecked, the harder it is to fix with stretching or conditioning.

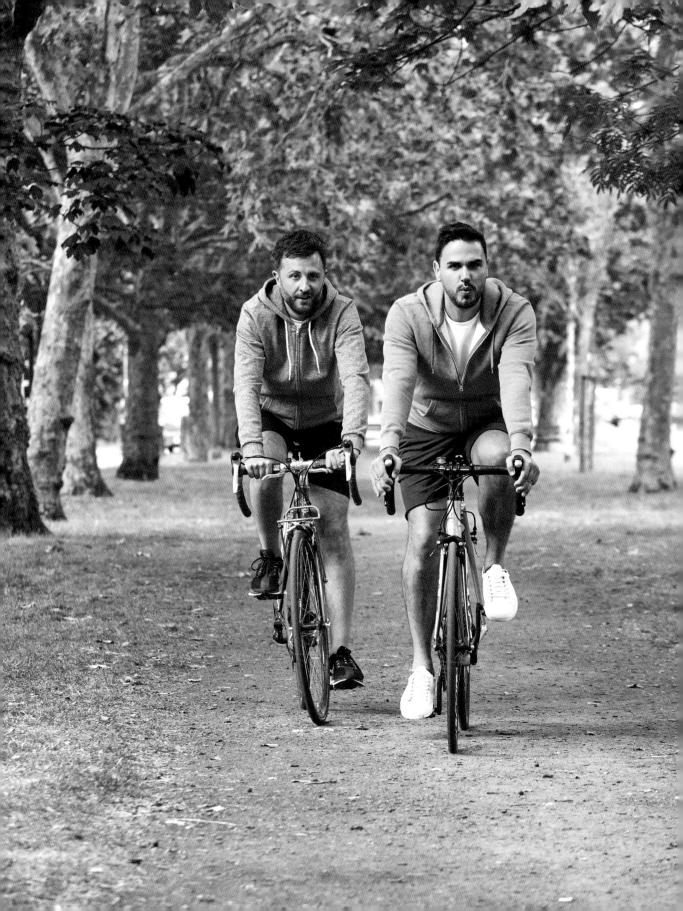

Exercise is also the number one way to look after your heart. Heart rate variability (HRV) is one of the best measurements of health, and also serves as a good indicator of how well your heart is working. Increasing your heart rate on a regular basis will help preserve the heart's health.

The best gift you can give your future self is that of agility and strength. Look after your body, as it's the only place you have to live.

Move daily

Make an effort to move on a daily basis, by including it in your daily routine. This may involve active hobbies, like going to the gym or a class, or could be simply walking to the bus stop twice a day. Just make choices that involve your body moving as much as possible.

A cool way to track this is with a smartphone or smartwatch. 10,000 steps is commonly used as a target for each day, and trackers for this can be found on almost all smartphones and smartwatches now. You could use a wall chart instead, and simply note down 30 minutes of active movement on a daily basis. Whatever you do, try to move every day.

Or try "exercise snacking": moving regularly for short periods throughout the day. Look for ways to introduce extra activity: Do you have a long work phone call scheduled? Could you do it while you go for a walk? Or if you have to travel to a meeting, can you incorporate some walking or cycling into the journey? If we have a meeting a few miles away and the weather's nice, we like to cycle, to help us keep active.

Exercise your heart weekly

Two or three times a week, do something that gets you breathing hard and your blood pumping. This could involve a run, a cycle, or simply a fast walk, but find a way to make it a bit strenuous. You need to be breathing hard enough that it's difficult to have a conversation. If you're able to talk to someone easily, you're not working hard enough.

Alternatively, if you're a gym goer, do some cardio, a high-intensity-interval-training (HIIT) workout, or simply lift weights faster! If you wear a smartwatch, then you're looking for an elevated heart rate as a sign that you are pushing your heart to work harder. Get that blood pumping to keep your heart fit. The heart is literally a muscle, and we want to make sure we keep it nice and strong.

Strengthen your muscles weekly

As we get older our muscles start to deteriorate. One of the best ways to fight this is to continually build muscle mass through strength training. The more muscle you have, the longer it will last.

We're not talking about building an Olympic body here—although it's up to you if you want to do that! We're talking about pushing your body to get strong and to build and retain muscle.

There are many ways to do this, but you might try cycling, rock climbing, yoga, Pilates, lifting light weights, or following fitness DVDs or YouTube videos—whatever works for you. Of course, you could use a personal trainer, too, although that can be quite an expensive option. There are plenty of strength-based classes at the gym or in local parks, or you can just do it at home.

And stretch . . .

Flexibility and mobility are two sides of the same coin. You want to be flexible enough that your joints and muscles can move through a large range of motion. We're not suggesting you should be able to do the splits, but being able to touch your toes is a good indicator of hamstring flexibility.

Ian has tight shoulders, and an area of focus for him has been working on raising his arms straight above his head. This might sound simple, but many of us have shoulders too tight to do this. And these limitations in flexibility can cause issues further down the line.

Mobility means that you have strength throughout your range of flexibility. So, in Ian's case, he doesn't just want to be able to reach his arms straight above his head, but also to be able to carry a weight safely through the whole range of motion. Your goal should be to improve your flexibility and mobility at the same time.

Regular stretching is great for building flexibility. If you're sitting in front of the TV on a rainy Sunday, then why not run through some gentle stretches at the same time? You can find loads of follow-along stretch videos on YouTube, and once you've learned them you won't need the videos any more.

Yoga is perhaps one of the best and most popular ways to build both flexibility and mobility. Pilates and barre work wonders, too, as does tai chi. Martial arts are also good choices, as are rock climbing, gymnastics, and calisthenics.

Another crucial part of improving mobility is breaking up tight muscle fibers. We all know what it feels like to have knots in our muscles, whether they're in our shoulders, back, or glutes. These are muscle fibers that have stuck together, and it's important to break them up to get good flexibility and range of motion. This can be done through massage, but not all of us can afford weekly massage sessions! The best way to do this for yourself is with an inexpensive foam roller—ideally one with little knobs on it. Find a follow-along video class where they'll show you how to use the roller to ease up tension in your muscles.

Find a form of exercise that you love

Whatever you choose to do, find an exercise that you love and make it part of your regular routine, aiming to exercise 3 to 5 times per week.

In the last few years, we have adopted a regular calisthenics and gymnastics schedule. We absolutely love it. We're not just lifting more weights, but at every session we achieve goals or levels that we would have never thought possible. When we started, we could barely do push-ups or pull-ups. Now we can perform them with ease, and we're working on handstands and doing cool flips on gymnastics rings. It makes every gym session fun!

Maybe you have a room at home where you can follow fitness class videos. Or maybe you prefer a gym class before or after work. We like to get our workouts done in the morning, so we can begin the day having worked out.

Commit to getting started by trying one type of exercise for a week. Make it a priority in your day—just like you've done with sleep. And see how much better you feel at the end of the week.

Find the right kind of exercise for you, as that's the only way you'll keep it up. Try different classes or home workouts until you find one that resonates with the way you want your body to move. You might fall in love with Zumba, or weight training. Or you might prefer to become a supple gymnast or Pilates master. Or perhaps 5 a.m. karate sessions in the park are more your thing.

Find a form of exercise you love and make it part of your regular routine, for a longer, happier life.

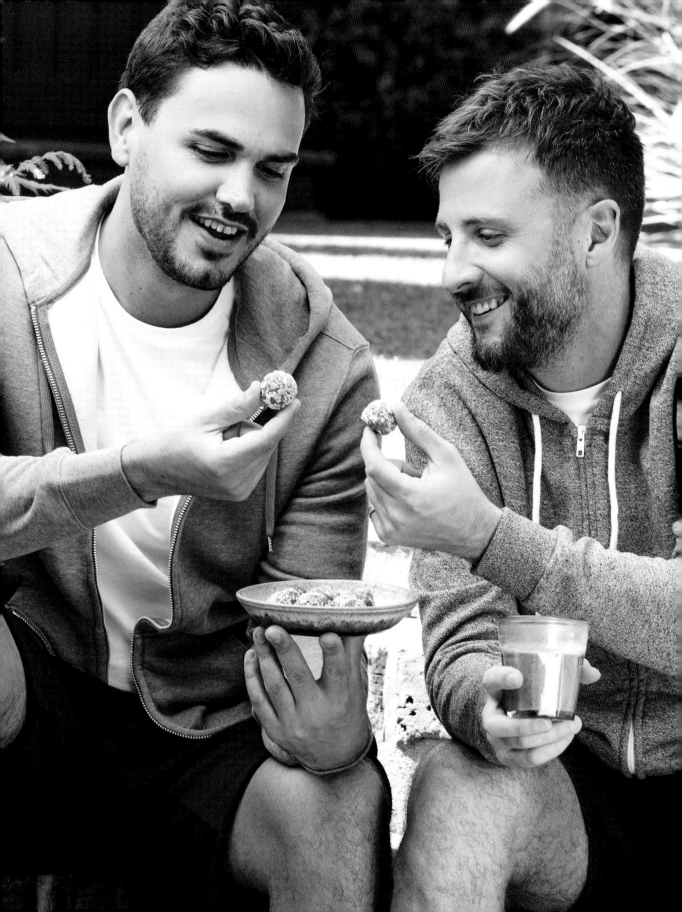

RELAX

Most of us are generally not that great at relaxing. We live busy, frantic lives running from task to task, constantly spinning plates. With no downtime, your brain is constantly in a state of stress. When you are overwhelmed with stress, your body is constantly in fight-or-flight mode, with high cortisol levels (cortisol is our body's stress hormone), which can lead to longer-term health consequences. Finding an opportunity each day to relax really helps to reduce stress, and promotes a more positive attitude to life.

Relaxing on a daily basis can give you a new default mode. Instead of being like a stretched elastic band, constantly under pressure, you'll find yourself existing in a more relaxed state of mind most of the time. If something stressful does happen, it's easier to deal with from a state of calm. It will also give you a more balanced view on life. You're less likely to lash out at those you love, and in difficult negotiations you will be more flexible. You'll find you sleep better, too, and might even find it benefits your exercise and general fitness. See? It all fits together beautifully!

Learn to meditate. Meditation is perhaps the most commonly talked about form of relaxation. Many people practice meditation or mindfulness on a daily basis to help quiet their minds. Apps like Headspace or Calm are great for this (we use both): you can practice meditating daily for 5, 10, 15, or even 30 minutes, and you'll experience benefits from the first session. If you prefer, attend meditation classes and learn the principles from a teacher, which you can then apply to your own practice. Forms of prayer work to quiet the mind, too, and both prayer and meditation have been linked to populations who live longer.

Focus on what you're grateful for, and let your internal voice thank the universe for that thing. Did you feel stressed? Probably not. It's hard, if not impossible, to be stressed while feeling grateful. Gratitude is a practice, almost like a muscle, that can be strengthened through daily exercise. Spend some time each day, either just in your mind or writing in a journal or on your phone, focusing on three things you are grateful for. This will help calm your mind, give you a more positive outlook, and reduce stress.

Factor in some "me time." We consider our morning workouts as "me time." They help clear our minds and give us a really positive boost for the day ahead. Me time is different for everyone—just think about what it is you like to do (which doesn't involve a screen) and find a way to do some of it every day. We love to cook, and even though it's what we do for our daily work, we still find cooking for ourselves in the evening to be relaxing. Other examples include reading, crossword puzzles, gardening, walking the dog, taking a long bath, yoga, or deep-breathing exercises. Even tidying the house can be a relaxing activity if you do it right. Whatever you do, find a way to get a bit of relaxing me-time into your day. Your body, mind, and soul will benefit.

LOVE YOURSELF

How can you love others if you don't first love yourself? Today's society often doesn't teach us to love ourselves, but rather to judge and compare ourselves with others. The psychological damage this does can be greater than anything the outside world presents us with.

Social media makes many of us feel like we aren't good enough. Fat-shaming or body-shaming is rife in today's world, and is a real form of emotional damage. We need to love ourselves and accept ourselves as we are right now.

Diet culture in general has us all comparing ourselves to those around us and wondering if they are better than us. Are we thin enough? Do we fit into those jeans? How do those squidgy bits look in the mirror?

It's true that there are correlational links between obesity and life expectancy, but it is thought that some of these links could be due to the pressure society places on those who are overweight, and the psychological harm that brings, rather than simply the amount of fat cells in a person's body.

Body neutrality literally means a feeling of neutrality toward your body. A blasé perspective about how your body looks. If you've been worrying about those love handles, or other bits of your body that you're not too keen on, then it's time to let that go. Equally, if you're very proud of your strong, round bum, or your big guns, then it's time to let that go, too. For more on this topic, check out Laura Thomas's awesome book *Just Eat It*.

In terms of your physical health, there are so many better things to focus on than your appearance, like overall strength and mobility (see page 29 for more on this). So, if you do want to focus on exercise, then focus on specific goals, rather than how you look. Aim to be able to touch your toes or run briskly up the stairs, rather than stressing about how you look in a bikini.

Overly focusing on the way our bodies look can lead to all kinds of disordered eating, such as extreme fasting, anorexia, binge comfort eating, yo-yo dieting, or bulimia.

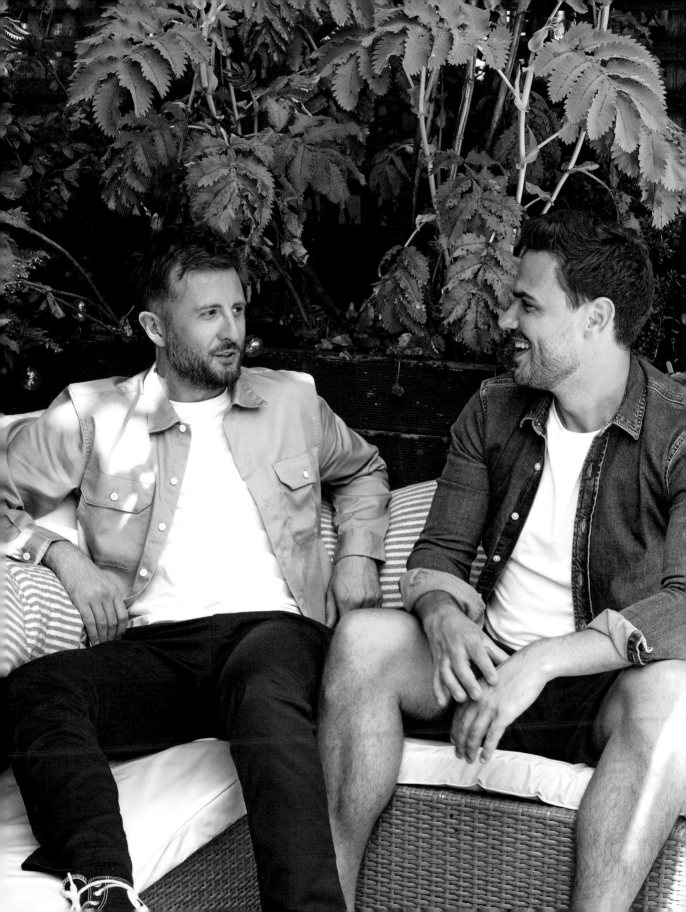

Your body is great at telling you when it's hungry and what nutrition it needs, so rather than focusing on what we "should" or "shouldn't" be eating, try to learn to focus on what your body is telling you it wants to eat.

Now this takes practice, and we don't mean "just eat all the sweets because you want to." It's unlikely that this is actually what your body is telling you it wants. Really think about your hunger levels and what your body is craving, while trying to overlook any addictive eating behaviors you may have learned.

Developing a more neutral attitude to the way your body looks will allow you to focus more on eating well and improving your overall health.

LOVE OTHERS

Feeling like you "belong" is crucial to a happy, healthy life. It could be a circle of friends or family members or a sports or book club, but being part of a tribe that you socialize with on a regular basis is really important to your health. Being around friends and family has been shown to have positive effects on stress levels, and being part of a social or family unit has been associated with longer lifespans.

This doesn't mean you need to suddenly become an extrovert out gallivanting every night. But it does mean spending time with others can have a positive effect on your life.

Make time for family and friends, even if you think you're too busy. Plan some fun activities that don't necessarily revolve around alcohol. Today, it's all too easy for fun to end up involving booze. That can be detrimental to other parts of your life and health. Set a date for enjoying some outdoor activities together, like hiking or playing mini-golf! Or catch up over movies and food, or a barbecue or dinner (why not cook some recipes from this book?). We're not saying you should go teetotal, but just don't let all your social activities involve drinking. Be social, spend time with family and friends, and make sure that social time has a positive impact on your day-to-day life.

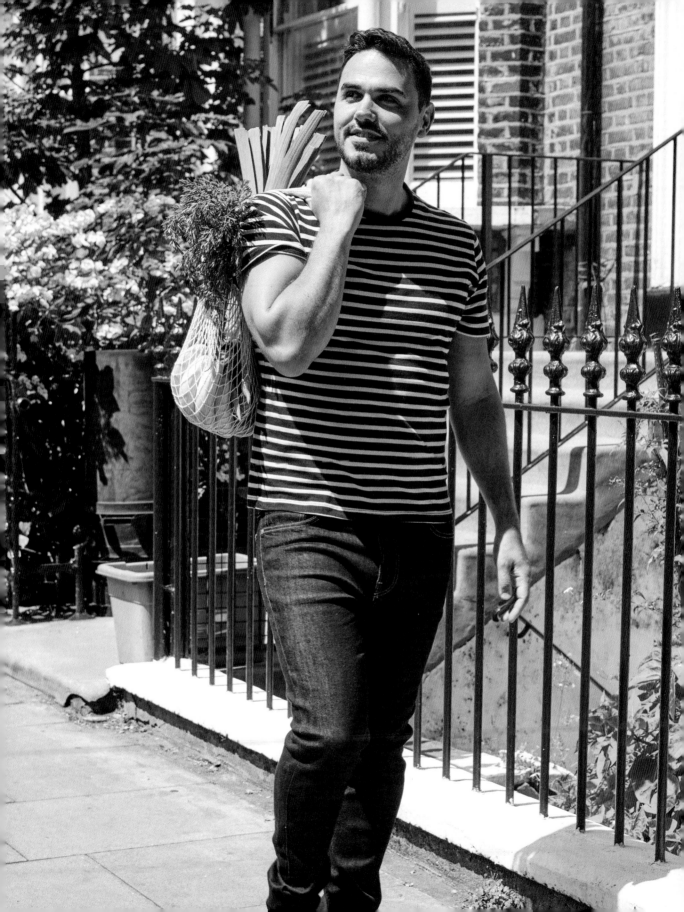

LIVE WITH PURPOSE

People with a core sense of purpose have been shown to live longer, healthier lives. The Japanese call this *ikigai*, which translates directly as "reason for being." Your driving purpose may be your career, or your religion; it may be community work, or caring for your family. Having a strong sense of purpose in life can help you remain happy and healthy.

This is core to our BOSH! beliefs as well. Both of us have a clear purpose— we are here to provide plant-based inspiration, knowledge, and recipes for people all around the world, and in this way do our bit to help tackle global climate change.

If there's a disconnect between what you do in your daily work or home life and what you believe, then that can have a real impact on your well-being. If you're unhappy at work, this can spill over into other parts of life. It may cause you to comfort eat, it may stop you from exercising, it may cause you to fall out with your family and friends. By contrast, if you're fulfilled by your work, then your relationships, personal routines, and habits are much easier to feel in control of.

This doesn't mean you have to leave your job to become the next Mother Teresa. Life's not like that! If your job enables you to look after and provide for your family, then that is a great life purpose in itself. Just make sure you are clear why you are doing what you are doing, and take satisfaction from that.

But now that you've taken this opportunity to think about your health and well-being, think about ways you could feel more fulfilled. If you resent Mondays and live for the weekend, then it might be time for a change. Could you retrain for a job that is more in line with what you love? Could you change aspects of your existing work and take on some new, more satisfying challenges? Could you volunteer in the community?

Let yourself choose things that matter to you, and those around you, and you'll find yourself living with purpose.

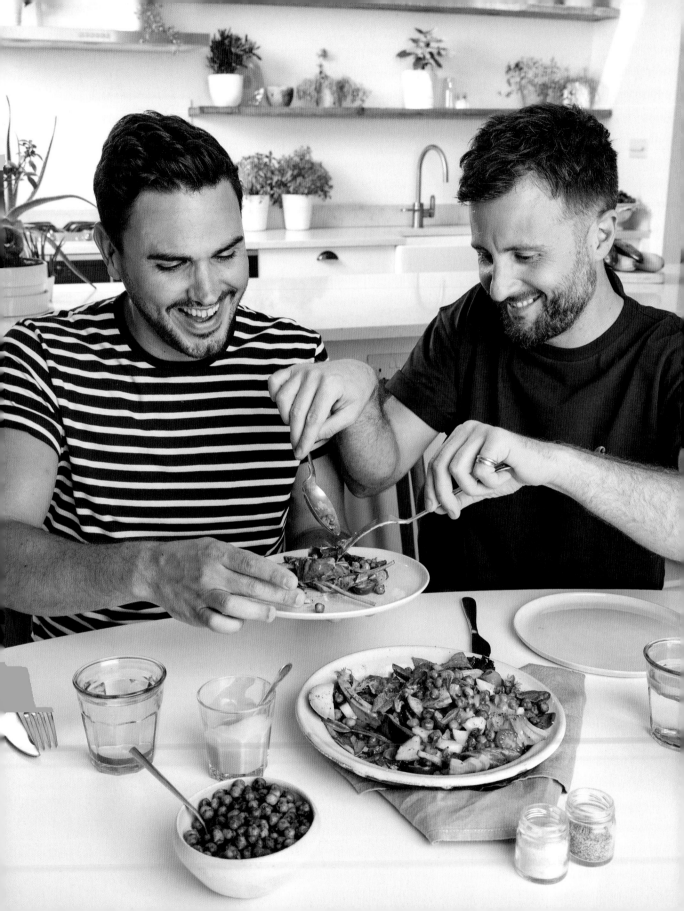

HOW TO EAT WELL

It's been said that we know more about the surface of the moon than we do the human digestive system. This may or may not be true, but there are certainly lots of different opinions about what we should and shouldn't eat.

By and large, though, there is plenty to point to a plant-based, or mostly plant-based, diet as being optimum for good health. And not just plant-based, but a way of eating that is based around mostly whole plant foods with varied colors, and avoiding foods that have been processed, such as white carbohydrates and sugars.

When you mention "vegan" or "plant-based," often everyone is suddenly an expert in nutrition and seriously concerned about your levels of protein or B12. For reference, on pages 49–52 we've included a breakdown of the different nutrients it is important to get on a plant-based diet, and the foods you can find them in.

The reality is that yes, it is possible to have nutritional deficiencies on a vegan diet (as it is on all diets), but it's easy to avoid if you do it right.

THE 5 GOLDEN RULES

You don't need to be an expert on nutrition to know how to eat well—healthy eating is for everyone. We've simplified our How to Eat Well principles into 5 easy-to-remember rules.

1. Follow the Rainbow Ratio: 50/25/25

2. Mix Up Your Plate

3. Eat Your Greens

4. Aim for 80/20

5. Get Your Vitamins

Follow these 5 basic principles, and you'll be on a healthy vegan diet for life.

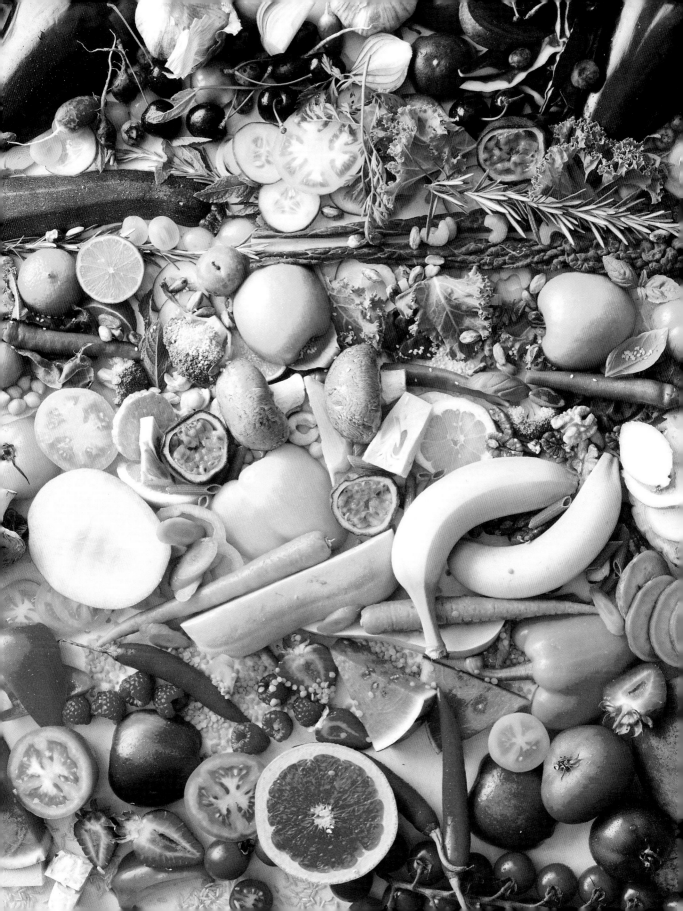

Follow the Rainbow Ratio: 50/25/25

Aim to eat about 50% fruits and veggies, 25% whole grains, and 25% proteins (legumes, nuts, and seeds). This is broadly in line with the Vegan Power Plate, the NHS Eatwell Plate, and the Canadian Food Plate (which leans toward plant-based eating).

The main issue is that the typical Western diet involves a very different ratio from this. It tends to revolve around large amounts of protein, and significantly lower amounts of fruits and veggies than we need in our day-to-day lives.

How often should we be eating these percentages? A dietician will tell you to eat a balanced plate at every single meal. That would mean that each meal would look something like the plate opposite. However, in real life this isn't always practical, since we'll often eat on the go or need to put together a meal quickly with whatever ingredients we have in the house. The rainbow ratio is a useful thing to know and bear in mind, but it's not a rule you have to stick to religiously. Just understand that when people talk about "a balanced diet," this is the ideal.

Aim for a mixed plate, making sure there are loads of fruits and veggies in your life on a daily basis, and that you are getting enough protein and grains.

And remember, a perfectly balanced, colorful plate doesn't have to mean a massive salad . . . it could equally mean a veggie lasagna or hearty chili.

Mix Up Your Plate

Our body thrives on plants. And variety. There are thousands of different plants, and many have varied health-promoting properties. Phytochemicals literally means chemicals from plants (phyto), and they collectively provide many of the important components that your body needs to function, repair, and grow.

The colors in veggies are caused by phytonutrients—natural chemicals that protect the plants from germs, bugs, the sun's harmful rays, and other things. Each color indicates an abundance of specific nutrients.

Eat a broad and varied range of foods and colors at every meal. Varying colors, textures, spices, and ingredients gives your body a broad range of health-promoting phytonutrients.

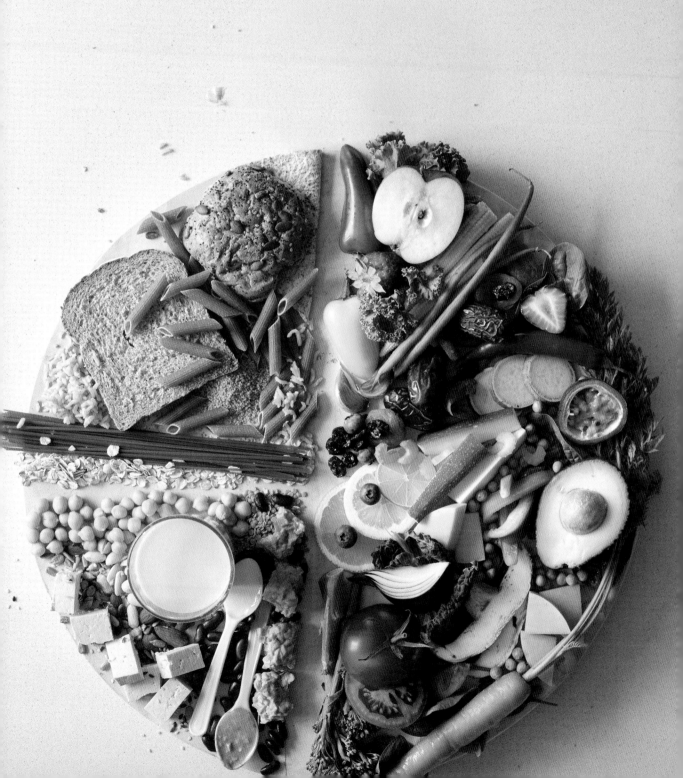

Green

Chlorophyll (which makes plants green) is packed with antioxidants and phytonutrients, and plants that contain it are a good source of fiber. Green phytonutrients are thought to help tissue healing and cell repair, detoxify the body, provide digestive enzymes, and boost the immune system. See page 46 for more on the benefits of going green.

  • **Sources:** broccoli, broccolini, spinach, kiwi fruit, zucchini, lettuce, and kale.

Red

Red fruits and veggies contain phytochemicals including lycopene and anthocyanins. These can only be found in plants and are health-promoting. They are thought to help reduce the risk of diabetes, heart disease, and stroke. They can improve skin quality, lower the risk of macular degeneration (thereby improving vision), and can soak up damaging free radicals.

  • **Sources:** raspberries, bell and chile peppers, tomatoes, strawberries, and watermelon.

White

White plants are colored by anthoxanthins and often also contain the phytonutrients allicin and quercetin. They can help keep bones strong, lower the risk of heart disease, help lower cholesterol, reduce inflammation, and balance hormones.

  • **Sources:** bananas, cauliflower, garlic, potatoes, and onions.

Purple and blue

Purple and blue fruit and vegetables are loaded with anthocyanins and resveratrol, which give them their deep rich color, and many of their health benefits. These fruit and veggies are thought to have anti-aging, anti-inflammatory, and disease-preventing properties.

  • **Sources:** blueberries, red cabbage, plums, eggplant (with skins on), and blackberries.

Yellow and orange

Yellow and orange fruit and vegetables are packed with carotenoids, giving them their carrot-like orange color. Sun-colored fruit and veggies also contain an abundance of vitamins and fiber.

- **Sources:** oranges, mangoes, sweet potatoes, carrots, and lemons.

Mix up your protein sources

Our body needs protein to help build and repair itself—so it's a crucial part of a balanced diet. And contrary to what many people believe, there is plenty of protein to be found in a plant-based diet.

Protein is made from a combination of twenty amino acids. Our body can make most of these itself, but there are nine that we need to get in our diet. These are called the "essential amino acids." "Complete proteins" contain all nine essential amino acids. Meat and animal products are all complete proteins, but there are only a handful of plant-based sources of protein that contain all nine amino acids, namely quinoa, buckwheat, and soy.

That doesn't mean you need to only eat those complete sources of plant protein. You just need to choose a wide range, so you eat all nine essential amino acids across your diet. For example, combining bread and peanut butter gives you all nine. Or any time you eat grains and beans together (such as rice and peas or chili with rice), you are getting all nine amino acids, too. You don't need to eat them all at one meal either—aim for variety across the day.

Eating a wide variety of different foods means you will easily hit your protein goals. As long as you are eating a varied diet and are getting enough calories, chances are you are eating enough protein. And even if you are a gym bunny or athlete, you can do that on a vegan diet, too—see our section on page 57 for more on eating plants for sports.

③ Eat Your Greens

Get as much green in your diet as you can. The fiber, vitamins, minerals, and phytochemicals in green vegetables can help lower cholesterol levels, improve vision, increase bone and bowel health, and provide nourishment for hair and skin. Eating green vegetables regularly can also help reduce the effects of environmental pollutants that accelerate aging, contribute to prevention of age-related memory loss, and improve cognitive and brain function. Anything dark green is packed with these micronutrients and phytochemicals that your body loves, so gorge on them!

- **Antioxidants and phytochemicals:** Eating leafy greens provides you with a wide range of these nutrients, which fight free-radical damage, improving your long-term health and lowering your risk of many diseases. Green phytonutrients in particular help with tissue healing, cell repair, and detoxifying the body; they also provide digestive enzymes, and boost the immune system.

- **Magnesium:** Chlorophyll is what gives plants their green color and at the center of the chlorophyll molecule is magnesium. Why is magnesium important? Well, it is needed for over 300 different enzymes in the body, including those that use and produce ATP—the energy currency of cells. But it is also crucial to cells that repair and destroy damaged cells, so it's really worth making sure your body has adequate magnesium to support those crucial processes. Some nuts such as almonds, Brazil nuts, and cashews, as well as pumpkin and sunflower seeds, also contain magnesium.

- **Vitamin C:** Green vegetables are a good source of vitamin C, a collagen-building antioxidant, which can help keep wrinkles, gray hair, and other signs of aging at bay. Greens are also thought to help fight acne, rosacea, and other skin conditions while strengthening the hair and reducing hair loss.

- **Lutein and indoles:** These are found in vegetables like bok choy, asparagus, and broccoli, and are thought to help strengthen bones and teeth and aid muscle recovery and tissue repair.

- **Fiber:** This helps eliminate accumulated toxins and waste in the colon, to prevent constipation. It plays an important role in maintaining healthy cholesterol levels and helps to stabilize blood glucose levels, too.

As you can see, the health benefits of green veggies are HUGE—so much so that it's worth getting a turbo charge of them into your body on a daily basis. There is no better way to start the day than with a giant green smoothie (see page 210), but aim to eat them throughout the day, too.

4 Aim for 80/20

Follow the 80/20 rule: 80% healthy and 20% naughty. It's OK from time to time to eat take-out meals or junk food (especially if it's home-cooked); just remember to balance it out with healthy and colorful foods the rest of the time.

Sometimes people forget that food is there to be enjoyed! Eating plays a huge part in our culture, in our family lives, in our sense of well-being. It's really important to find a way of eating that fits in with your life and makes you feel happy and relaxed, and that is sustainable for you in the long term.

Some people say "all things in moderation," some people say "don't overthink it," but both essentially mean the same thing. You're much more likely to stick to a new way of eating if it is flexible and works with your lifestyle, rather than if it's rigid or restrictive. Find a way that works for you so you never feel like you're missing out.

5 Get Your Vitamins

Nutrition isn't something that people are generally taught in school—unless we're faced with a problem or an illness we tend to just get on with things. And yet, research shows that large swaths of people are deficient in certain key nutrients. Common deficiencies that are prevalent across the UK population are: iron, iodine, vitamin D, vitamin B12, calcium, vitamin A, and magnesium.

Some of these deficiencies, like that of B12 or vitamin D, are more common in vegans. Therefore, it makes sense to take responsibility for getting the right nutrients into your body.

Some people find it helpful to take a multivitamin on a daily (or nearly daily) basis. If you are unsure which type to go for, ask your doctor. This, plus making sure you are getting enough vitamin D and B12, is a good place to start.

We both take a daily multivitamin. We try to make sure we have lots of sources of B12 in our diet through fortified milks, yeast extract, and nutritional yeast—but supplements are available. We also boost our omega-3 fatty acids (known as EPA and DHA, which are important for heart health) with a plant-based, algae-derived supplement. And if it's not sunny we have a little vitamin D spray that we carry around with us.

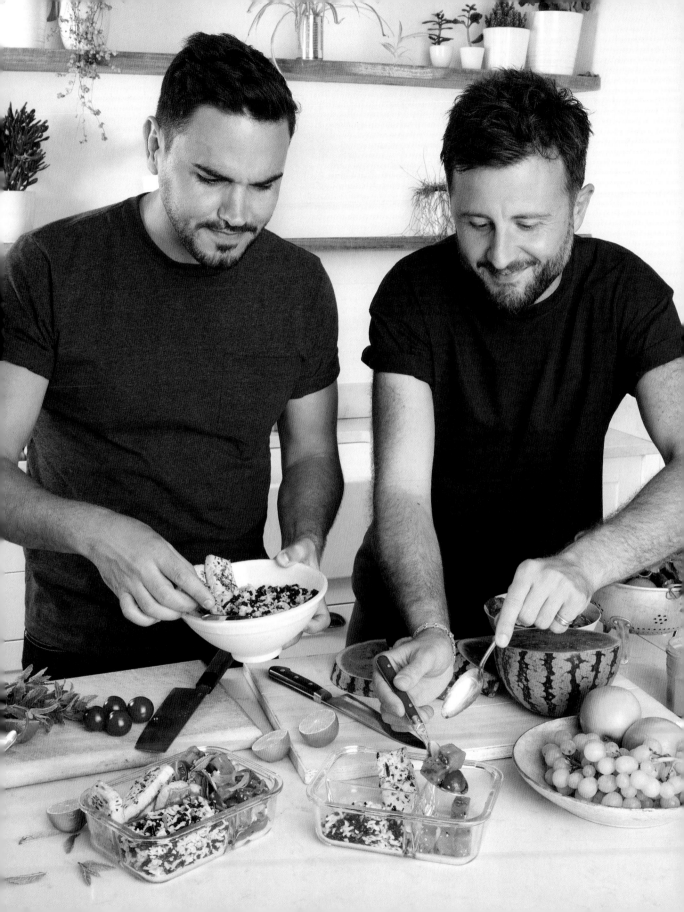

KEY NUTRIENTS

As humans, we don't eat vitamins and minerals, we eat food. So we think it's more helpful to think about the principles of eating a balanced diet rather than trying to eat specific foods for specific nutrients. That said, it is sometimes useful to have a point of reference, particularly if you discover you are deficient in a nutrient, so you can dial up the amounts of that nutrient you are getting in your food.

If you're making our recipes and following our five easy nutrition rules (page 40), you should have a good level of nutrition, but do check in with a doctor or dietician from time to time for peace of mind.

We are firm believers that we should all be reading up a little more on nutrition, and taking responsibility for our own dietary health. So, on the following pages is a reference for many of the most important nutrients to consume on a plant-based diet.

Vitamin B12

Vitamin B12 is important for red blood cell function and our central nervous system as well as the process of releasing energy from food. Some people can develop vitamin B12 deficiency (pernicious anemia) if they don't have enough in their diet, which can cause serious symptoms, starting with tiredness, a lack of energy, muscle weakness, or even memory issues. If you feel you might be experiencing any of these symptoms, consult your doctor for a blood test. B12 is common in meat, but isn't found naturally in plant products. This means that it is typically advisable to supplement, either via a pill or by consuming B12-fortified foods—most nondairy milks are now fortified with vitamin B12.

- Fortified nondairy milks
- Fortified breakfast cereals
- Yeast extract, such as Marmite, which has been fortified with vitamin B12

Vitamin D

Many people in the northern hemisphere are low in vitamin D, since our body makes it by being exposed to the sun. It's vital for good health, and for keeping bones, teeth, and muscles healthy. It also helps regulate the amount of calcium in our body. Most doctors recommend adults take a vitamin D supplement, especially in the colder months, as it can be hard to get enough from food alone. Some good vegan sources include:

- Fortified spreads, breakfast cereals, and nondairy milks
- Mushrooms, particularly if they are vitamin D-fortified

Omega-3 and omega-6 fatty acids

These two types of fats, also known as polyunsaturated fats, are needed by our bodies, but our body can't create them. This means we need to get them from our diets. It's not just the amounts of these fats, but also the ratio that we have in our body that's important. Omega-3 is a little harder to get on a vegan diet, which sometimes means we may have a ratio that is tipped too far toward the omega-6 end of the scale. To get good amounts of omega-3s into your diet, make sure you are eating the following:

- Ground flaxseeds, flaxseed oil
- Chia seeds
- Walnuts
- Canola oil
- Seaweed (and algae)
- Edamame
- Kidney beans
- Soy-based foods, including tofu

Iodine

This is a key part of healthy thyroid function, keeping your body's metabolism and cell function working properly. Seaweed is a rich source of iodine, although it can be difficult to know how much you're getting, and you could be at risk of having too much, so a supplement is usually recommended.

- Fortified nondairy milks
- Seaweed, including kelp, nori, and sea vegetables
- Cereals and grains

Iron

An important part of red blood cell function, iron helps ensure oxygen is carried around your body correctly. Some people's iron levels can be low, particularly if they are an athlete or a woman with heavy periods. If you think you may be anemic, consult your doctor and get your blood checked, then adjust your diet accordingly, including more iron-rich foods and avoiding foods that contain iron inhibitors like phytates and polyphenols, found in grains and beans, the tannins in tea, and some spices such as chiles. Good plant-based sources of iron include:

- Fortified breakfast cereals
- Nuts
- Dried fruit, including dates, figs, and prunes
- Most dark green leafy vegetables, such as watercress and kale
- Sweet potatoes
- Peas
- Tofu
- Artichokes
- Pumpkin and pumpkin seeds
- Dark chocolate

Calcium

Calcium is an important part of a healthy diet. We need it to build strong bones and teeth. It also helps with healthy blood function and blood clotting. It goes hand in hand with vitamin D (see opposite), which helps us to absorb calcium. Good plant-based sources include:

- Fortified nondairy milks, creams, and yogurts
- Tofu
- Leafy vegetables, such as watercress and kale
- Nuts, especially Brazil nuts
- Green leafy vegetables, such as broccoli, cabbage, and okra (but not spinach)
- Dried fruit, such as figs, raisins, prunes, and apricots
- Seeds, especially sesame seeds (and tahini)
- Fortified breads

Magnesium

An essential nutrient that assists in hundreds of processes in your body, including repairing and regenerating cells and providing energy, and regulating blood-sugar levels. It is even thought to help with anxiety. Luckily it's plentiful in:

- Avocados
- Chard
- Spinach
- Black beans
- Bananas
- Figs
- Almonds
- Pumpkin seeds
- Dark chocolate

Vitamin A

This supports your immune system, helps maintain good eyesight, and also helps keep skin healthy. Do be aware that you don't want to have too much vitamin A, as large quanties can be harmful (especially if you are pregnant). It's absolutely possible to get all the vitamin A you need from your diet, but if you're concerned, ask your doctor. Beta-carotene is converted into vitamin A in the body, so some great plant-based sources include:

- Yellow and red vegetables, such as carrots, butternut squash, pumpkin, sweet potatoes, and red peppers, as well as yellow fruit like mango, papaya, and apricots.
- Kale
- Spinach

Zinc

Zinc helps regulate and improve the functioning of the immune system as well as assisting in making new cells throughout the body. You can find it in:

- Leafy green vegetables
- Sprouted seeds and beans
- Seeds

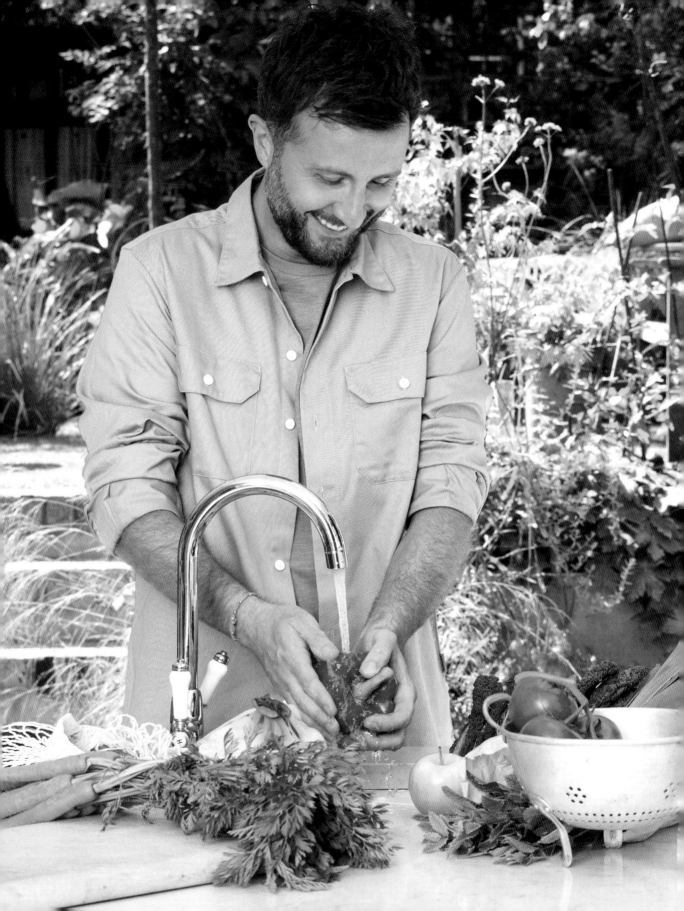

LOSING FAT

Many people turn to plant-based eating as a way to lose fat. We've heard countless stories of people who turned vegan and dropped weight quickly, and for good.

A healthy plant-based diet has a lower caloric density than other ways of eating, while being higher in fiber. A whole foods plant-based diet is also likely to be lower in fat. That means that you can feel fuller for longer, due to all the plants you are consuming, but the amount of calories is actually lower.

Conversely, we know vegans for whom the opposite is true. If you are eating plenty of oils in the form of avocados, vegan cheeses, and nut butters, then you will be taking on board many more calories. This is one of the reasons that some vegans try to follow an oil-free or low-fat plant-based diet. And if you are eating lots of refined carbs and sugars, they can potentially stimulate, rather than satisfy, your appetite.

Likewise, if you are following what is affectionately known as a "junk food vegan" diet, then you are unlikely to lose fat, and more likely to gain it. That way of eating involves lots of high-calorie fatty foods, lots of processed fake meats and white carbohydrates, and not enough plants and fiber. So, just following a vegan diet isn't enough if you want to lose fat.

Eating mindfully can also help with managing weight. Rather than eating automatically, listen to your body and eat only when you're hungry. Drinking plenty of water can also help with this. And remember, it can take up to 20 minutes for your brain to realize your stomach is full, so eat slowly and spend time savoring every mouthful. Eat at the table rather that in front of the TV, and limit distractions during mealtimes. Focus on what you're eating and your enjoyment of your meal.

Our best advice is to stop thinking about your weight completely, as hard as that may sound. Stop thinking about losing fat and start making some small changes toward a long-term healthier lifestyle. If you follow our 5 Golden Rules on how to eat well on pages 40–47, and adopt our principles for how to live well on pages 23–37, over the next few months you will feel healthier and more agile following a colorful, varied diet.

Focus on getting 7 to 9 hours of sleep each night (see page 24) and aim to hit a healthy "move goal" every day (see page 28). Combining our 10,000 steps a day with a healthy diet—like the recipes in this book—80% of the time, has allowed us to shape up, build muscle, and feel the healthiest we've ever felt, at the age of 35.

In summary:

- Eat mostly unprocessed, whole plant-based foods
- Sleep well (avoid caffeine in the afternoon)
- Be active
- Slow down your eating and chew more—eat mindfully
- Stay hydrated—make water your drink of choice
- Avoid sugar

Following these simple lifestyle principles should be more than enough to help you maintain a healthy body weight. However, if you're still set on losing fat, here are our top tips for a leaner lifestyle.

Watch your calories

Although there is a bit more to it than simply burning calories, the calories-in, calories-out equation does largely work as a guide to maintaining a healthy weight. But for fat loss, what we eat is almost more important than exercise. As Henry's fiancée likes to remind him, "abs are made in the kitchen."

The recommended daily intake of calories to maintain a healthy weight are 2,500 for an average man, and 2,000 for an average woman. Adopt a regular exercise routine and make sure that you take these recommendations into account in your daily calorie intake.

② Consider your relationship with food

Rather than the equations around calories failing us, often an unhealthy relationship with food can be at the root of overeating. We all sometimes use food to soothe or distract us from other problems. Feelings of guilt and shame around these behaviors are common, which can in turn lead to a binge-purge cycle with food. If you find yourself snacking or overeating when you're feeling angry, tired, sad, bored, or lonely, then try to find another way to lift yourself out of that state. Go for a walk, call a friend, have a bath–whatever it is that will make yourself feel better and distract you from reaching for food (see page 32 for more on the importance of relaxation). But if this is a more significant issue or pattern for you, it's important to seek professional help.

③ Avoid fad diets or transformations

Don't simply reach for "raw vegan" or "alkaline" diets, or paleo, keto, low-carb diets, just because they're the latest flavor of the month. They may work in the short term, but encourage a disordered approach to eating, which is hard to sustain in the long term, and are likely to cause you to fall off the wagon, and potentially put all the weight back on again. Make good food choices consistently over time, incorporate healthy eating into your regular lifestyle, and you will see positive results–and sustain them for life.

A QUICK WORD ON MACRONUTRIENTS

As we've said, by and large we like to think about food as food. We don't eat macronutrients, we eat food! So trying to break foods down into protein foods, carbohydrate foods, or fatty foods is kind of impossible. All foods contain combinations of these macronutrients anyway. Once you start to tailor your diet around healthy whole foods, colorful plants, protein-packed legumes, nuts, and seeds and whole grains, you'll find you eat healthily without having to count calories or macros. If you are looking for more on protein, then skip to our "Building Muscle" section opposite.

BUILDING MUSCLE

There are plenty of professional athletes who follow a plant-based diet, so you, too, can use vegan foods to fuel an athletic lifestyle and/or to build muscle mass. Our core advice here is the same as ever—eat whole foods! Many athletes even say that they find their body recovers from exercise more quickly while on a plant-based diet.

Someone who is looking to gain weight or build muscle will obviously need to consume more calories than they use. Carefully estimate the increase in calories you will need (a professional should be able to help you with this) and then use the calorie counts in this book to find meals to achieve your goals. You can top up your daily intake with smoothies, as well as prioritizing high-calorie snacks like nuts, nut butters, and avocados.

Stay hydrated, and before and after training aim to get plenty of complex carbs into your body, to give you maximum energy for the workout and to aid recovery afterward. Aim for high-quality, lower-GI carbohydrates and grains like brown rice and quinoa rather than refined carbohydrates like pasta or bread. You might choose to increase your fat intake in order to achieve higher calorie counts, but you should still avoid saturated fats where possible.

Our body particularly needs enough protein when aiming to build muscle, as this is what the body uses to heal and repair itself (see page 44). But you can get plenty on a plant-based diet. Make tofu, tempeh, legumes, nuts, seeds, and whole grains a staple. There are also plenty of healthy plant-based protein powders, such as pea protein or hemp protein, that can increase your daily protein intake, too. However, do be aware that increasing protein isn't necessarily a great thing to do—some studies have shown that too much protein can be detrimental to our health.

All the recipes in this book are labeled clearly with protein and fat quantities per portion, and recipes that are a good source of protein are clearly labeled. We've recommended a few to get started with on page 60.

It's important, if you are looking for weight gain, to work with a sports dietician who will use evidence-based advice and techniques to help you achieve your goals, whatever the sport or discipline you're interested in.

THE BOSH! HEALTHY VEGAN RECIPES...

. . . are easy, quick, healthy, and delicious

We love creating great-tasting vegan food and sharing it with you. Millions of people sharing and cooking our meals all over the world is what gets us up in the morning. We've put all of that love of flavor into the recipes in this book. As always, our recipes are bulletproof, having been tested multiple times. And they're quick! Almost every dish can be on the table in under 30 minutes.

. . . have been fine-tuned for your health

We've designed them in line with the best available medical wisdom and dietary guidelines. We're not trying to sell you quirky powders, esoteric ingredients, or unpronounceable imported foodstuffs.

Because our recipes are plant-based, they are naturally healthier. A plant-based diet, particularly one high in fiber and low in fat, is a really good way to eat. So your easy way to a healthy diet is to eat the recipes in this book! Eat a mix of all the recipes and you'll be in a great place.

. . . are in line with trusted dietary recommendations

The recipes in this book have been designed with various healthy eating principles in mind. First is the 50/25/25 plate, which we've covered already in our 5 Golden Rules on page 40. These recipes are mixed plates, with a good balance of proteins, fats, and carbohydrates on each plate. And they are, broadly speaking, made up of the right balance of different food groups.

This way of designing a plate corresponds with various, well-trusted sources of dietary best practice, including the NHS Eatwell Plate and the Canadian government's Food Plate. Our recipes are also designed in line with an easily achievable interpretation of Dr. Greger's Daily Dozen, which recommends the types of foods vegans should eat on a daily basis.

. . . are balanced in line with UK guidelines

We've nutritionally analyzed the recipes, and tweaked and tinkered with them, so they are in line with best practices from a dietary perspective. We've worked with an HCPC-registered dietician to get the portion sizes and macronutrient breakdown just right. We've also used the nutritional traffic light system that's applied to supermarket foods to ensure that our recipes are healthy: all our recipes fall within the green—or a little bit orange occasionally—part of the spectrum. We've taken care to ensure none of them are high in saturated fat, and we've worked hard to avoid using too much salt, sugar, and fat.

They are all high in flavor, without being high in anything bad for you. But don't just take our word for it—try them for yourself. And we'd love to hear from you once you've tried it!

Our recipes are also generally low in processed foods. If we are using a processed carbohydrate (for example, pasta) we've typically gone for the higher-fiber and lower-GI whole grain version.

We've catered to dietary requirements

To help with any specific plans you may be following, we've included calorie counts per portion for each recipe. For ease, we've also labeled which recipes are:

LOW FAT

LOW SUGAR

FULL OF FIBER

PROTEIN PACKED

If you're looking for low-fat and oil-free recipes, then simply choose the recipes marked as low in fat and remove the oil. You can use water or vegetable stock for frying instead of oil, if you wish.

FANTASTIC FEASTS FOR EVERYONE

Everyone is different and healthy food means different things to each of us. Whatever you're after, we've got you covered. This whole book is healthy and packed with planty of goodness. But if you want something specific, look no further. Whether it's protein, low sugar, gluten-free, whole foods plant-based, or just meaty vegan food that you're after, these are our top picks for you.

HIGH FIBER

Fiber is one of the most important things for us all to get in our diet. It's good for our gut and energy levels and helps us maintain a healthy weight. These dishes are all packed with plant fiber.

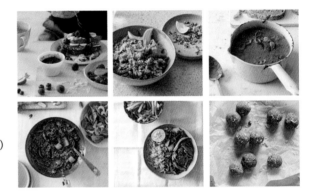

Healthy Banana French Toast (page 230)
Nasi Goreng (page 75)
Indian Spiced Tomato Soup (page 86)
Braised Jack Chili (page 125)
Feijoada & Slaw (page 127)
Bakewell BOSH! Balls (page 198)

HIGH PROTEIN

If you're looking to smash workouts and refuel your body, then these high-protein recipes are what you need. Get them in before or after the gym for maximum impact.

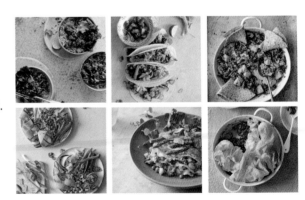

Total Protein Chili (page 141)
Ultimate Veg Tacos (page 67)
Healthy Saag Paneer (page 73)
Super Sushi Salad (page 117)
Salad Lasagna (page 154)
Meaty Mushroom Pie (page 163)

GLUTEN-FREE

If you're looking to avoid gluten, these recipes are all naturally and deliciously gluten-free.

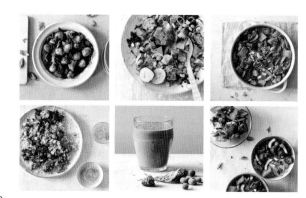

Puttanesca Potato Stew (page 70)
Zingy Watermelon Salad (page 93)
Sunny Sri Lankan Curry (page 153)
Jerk Jackfruit Salad 'n' Beans (page 118)
Green Goddess Smoothie (page 210)
Garden Party Breakfast Bowl (page 232)

LOW SUGAR

We all know that eating too much sugar is bad for our health. We've kept all the recipes in this book pretty low on sugar, but here are a handful of our favorite low-sugar recipes.

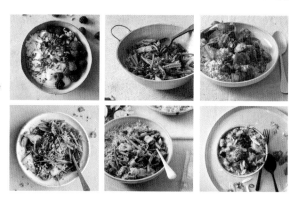

Summer Berry Granola Bowl (page 229)
Spicy Sichuan-Style Shiitake Stir-Fry (page 79)
Mixed Veg Katsu Curry (page 83)
Satay Salad (page 101)
Goan-Style Curry (page 144)
Legendary Rendang (page 175)

LOW FAT

One of the best things about eating a balanced plant-based diet is that it's naturally low in fat, while still being tasty and satisfying. These recipes are all proudly low in fat and high in flavor!

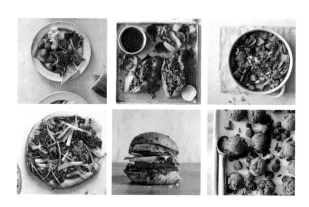

Mexi Breakfast (page 219)
BBQ Sloppy Jackets (page 138)
Sunny Sri Lankan Curry (page 153)
Hoisin Jackfruit Pizza (page 172)
Not-That-Naughty Burger with Frisbee Fries (page 178)
Banana Berry Ice Cream (page 204)

LOWER CALORIE

If you're looking to keep your calories in check then these recipes are all under 500 calories per portion.

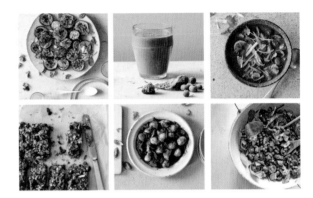

BOSH! Burnt Eggplant (page 98)
Green Goddess Smoothie (page 210)
Tom Yummo Soup (page 80)
BOSH! Bars (page 224)
Puttanesca Potato Stew (page 70)
Middle Eastern Spiced Chickpea Salad
  (page 104)

EAT THE RAINBOW

Eating the rainbow is all about getting as much color into your body as possible. These recipes are packed with colorful plants and health-giving phytonutrients.

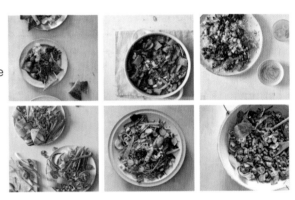

Mexi Breakfast (page 219)
Sunny Sri Lankan Curry (page 153)
Jerk Jackfruit Salad 'n' Beans (page 118)
Super Sushi Salad (page 117)
Rainbow Stir-Fry (page 108)
Middle Eastern Spiced Chickpea Salad
  (page 104)

VEGGIE MEAT

Are you looking to cook dishes that are plant-based, but replicate the taste or heartiness of eating meat? We've got you covered! These dishes are protein-packed and meaty-tasting!

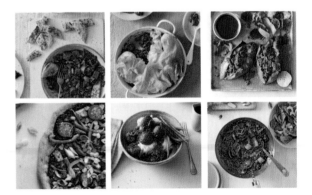

EmJ's Hearty Hotpot (page 150)
Meaty Mushroom Pie (page 163)
BBQ Sloppy Jackets (page 138)
Texas BBQ Pizza (page 168)
Meatballs with Mash & Gravy (page 182)
Braised Jack Chili (page 125)

WHOLE FOODS PLANT-BASED

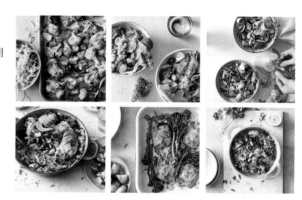

Eating whole foods plant-based means you'll be eating unprocessed and unrefined foods that are low in fat. With these recipes, you can replace the oil with water if you like.

Cat's Curryflower (page 148)
Niçoise Salad (page 97)
Thai Tempeh Salad (page 120)
Green Shakshuka (page 112)
"Salmon" Tofu Steaks (page 111)
Hearty, Herby Stew (page 128)

HOT & SPICY

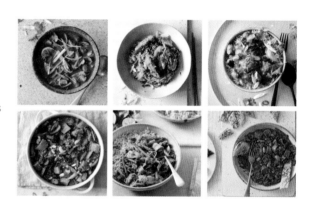

Eating the rainbow isn't just about color—getting spices into your diet is crucial, too. These dishes are perfect for adding that fiery punch of chile and aromatic goodness to your life.

Tom Yummo Soup (page 80)
Crispy, Sticky Tofu with Rice (page 186)
Legendary Rendang (page 175)
Sunny Sri Lankan Curry (page 153)
Goan-Style Curry (page 144)
EmJ's Hearty Hotpot (page 150)

PARTY FOOD

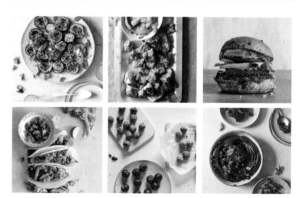

Eating well is about enjoying your food. If you've got your squad coming over, these dishes are perfect for sharing. From little nibbles to finger foods, this is what we'd serve you at a BOSH! house party!

BOSH! Burnt Eggplant (page 98)
Crispy Tofu Satay Bites (page 84)
**Not-That-Naughty Burger with Frisbee
  Fries** (page 178)
Ultimate Veg Tacos (page 67)
BOSH! Balls (pages 198–189)
Banana & Chocolate Mousse (page 197)

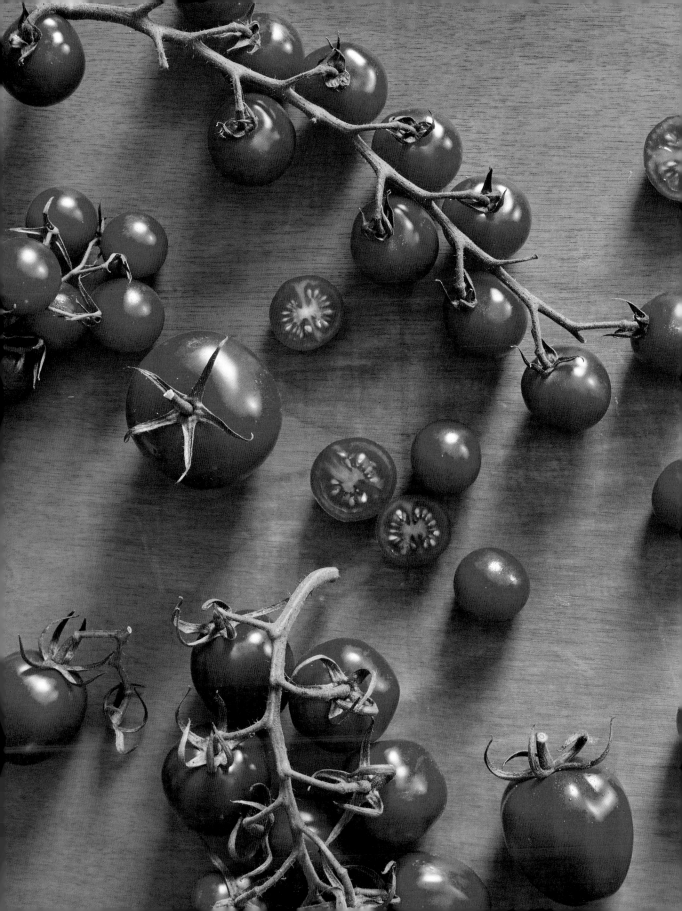

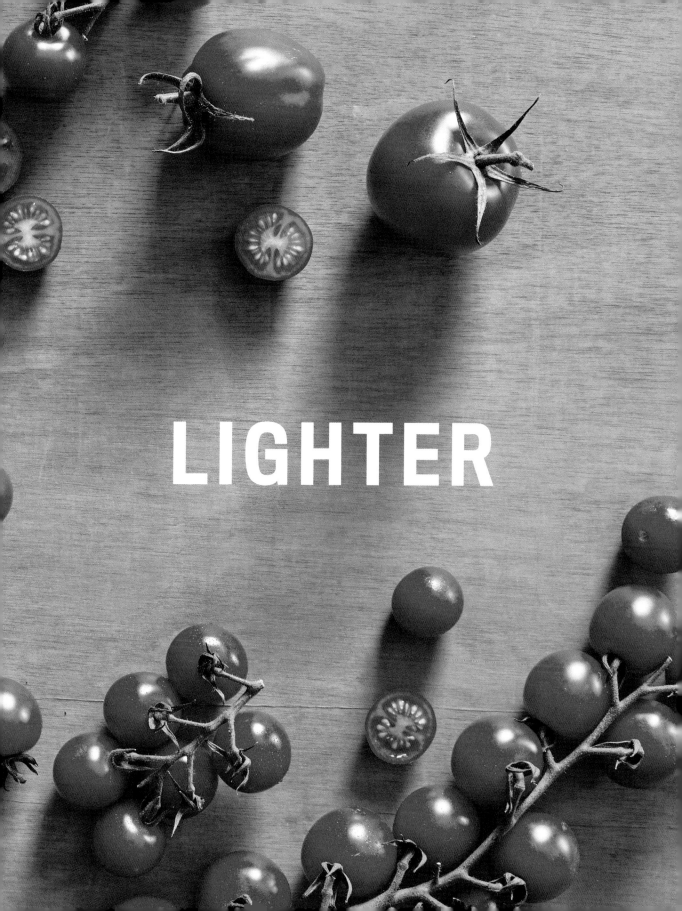

LIGHTER

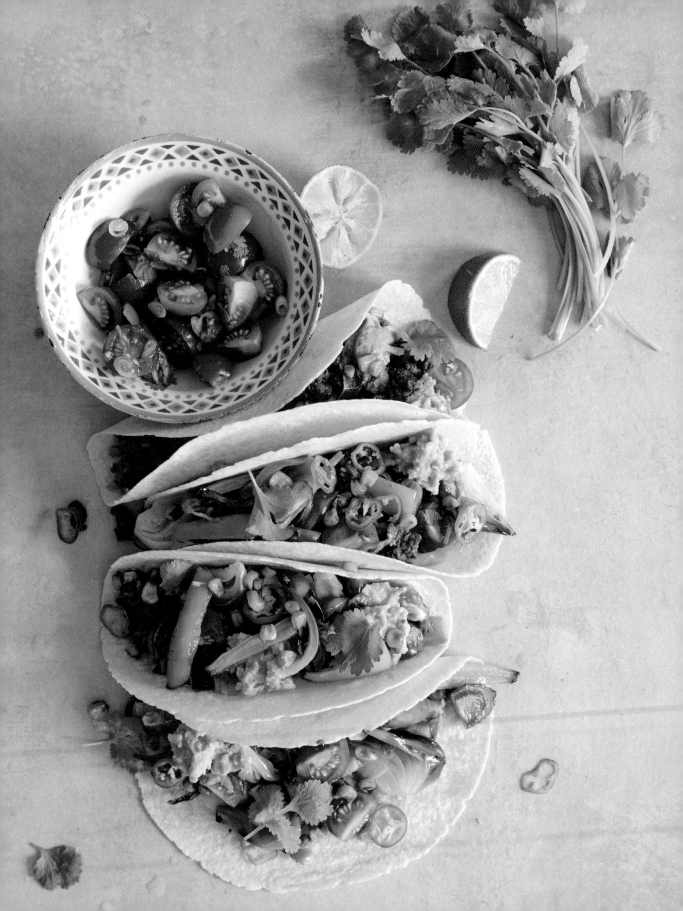

ULTIMATE VEG TACOS

SERVES 4

FOR THE ROASTED PEPPERS

1 red onion
2 orange bell peppers
1 tbsp olive oil
salt and black pepper

FOR THE ROASTED CORN

1 (7 oz) can corn (no salt added)
½ tsp smoked paprika
½ tbsp olive oil

FOR THE BANGIN' BLACK BEANS

2 garlic cloves
1 (14 oz) can black beans
1 tbsp olive oil
½ tsp ground cinnamon
½ tsp ground cumin

FOR THE SIMPLE SALSA

2 oz cherry tomatoes
1 scallion
¼ cup fresh cilantro leaves
¼ tsp chili powder
½ lime

FOR THE AVO' TANG

1 ripe avocado
1 lime

TO SERVE

½ fresh green chile
2 limes
8 small corn tortillas
½ cup fresh cilantro leaves

These tacos are a feast for the eyes! We love the combination of colors, textures, and flavors—it has everything you could wish for in a meal. With the simple salsa and avocado tang, it also works really well as a side with lots of dishes and salads.

PREHEAT OVEN TO 350°F | LINE 2 SHEET PANS WITH PARCHMENT PAPER | FINE GRATER OR MICROPLANE | SMALL SAUCEPAN

First, roast the peppers | Peel, halve, and cut the red onion into scant ¼-inch-thick strips | Halve, core, and cut the peppers into scant ¼-inch-thick slices | Put the onion and pepper in a bowl, drizzle over the olive oil, add a pinch each of salt and pepper, and toss to combine | Spread out on one of the lined baking sheets, put in the oven, and bake for 25–30 minutes

Get the roasted corn in the oven | Drain and rinse the corn, pat dry with paper towels, then tip the kernels into a bowl with the smoked paprika and stir to combine | Sprinkle over a little salt and pepper, tip the corn onto the second sheet pan, put the pan in the oven, and roast for 30 minutes, stirring halfway through | Take both pans out of the oven, drizzle the corn with the oil, and set to one side

Meanwhile, make the black beans | Peel and grate the garlic | Drain and rinse the beans, reserving some of the water from the can, tip them into a bowl, and mash with a fork | Heat the olive oil in the small saucepan over medium heat | Add the garlic and stir for 30 seconds | Stir in the cinnamon and cumin | Add the black beans and stir to combine, adding the water to loosen the mixture | Taste and season to perfection with salt and pepper

Make the simple salsa | Quarter the tomatoes | Trim and thinly slice the scallion | Roughly chop the cilantro | Put the chili powder in a bowl, squeeze in the lime juice and stir | Stir in the tomatoes, scallion, and cilantro, and set to one side

Make the avo' tang | Halve and carefully pit the avocado by tapping the pit firmly with the heel of a knife so that it lodges in the pit, then twist and remove | Halve the lime | Scoop the avocado flesh into a bowl, squeeze in the lime juice, and mash with a fork to a textured cream

Lay all the elements of your Ultimate Veg Tacos on the table | Trim and thinly slice the chile | Cut the limes into wedges | Spoon a layer of beans and roasted pepper and onion onto each tortilla | Spoon over some avo' tang and simple salsa | Sprinkle with roasted corn, garnish with cilantro leaves and chile, add a squeeze of lime, and serve

203 KCAL | LOW SUGAR | FULL OF FIBER | PROTEIN PACKED

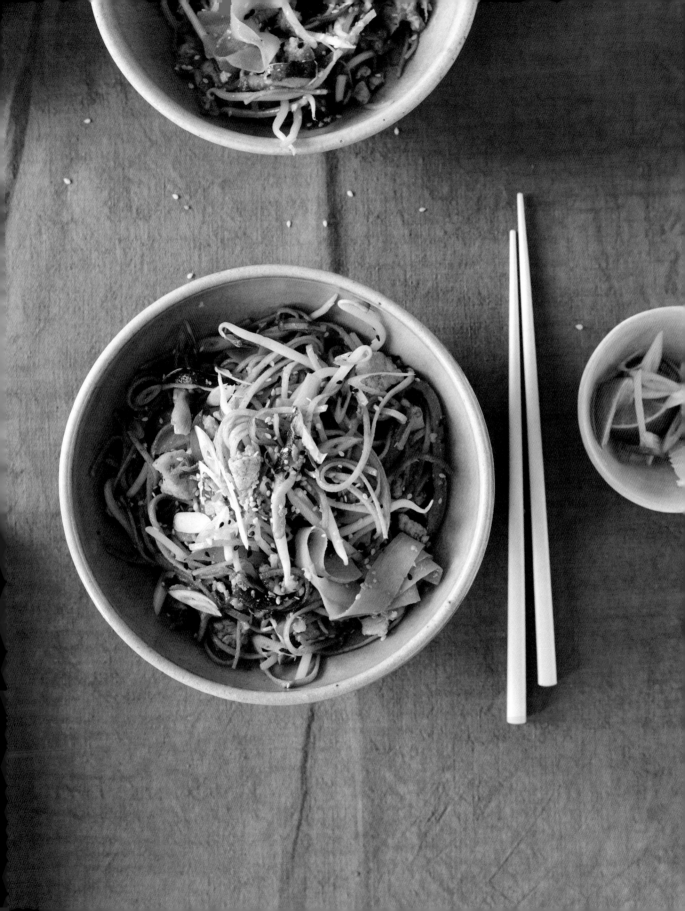

TOFU YAKI BOSH!

Yakisoba is one of our favorite noodle dishes, and this healthy version is brimming with goodness. Bean sprouts are a great source of protein, vitamin C, and folate, and add a satisfying crunch to dishes. Sesame seeds are a source of calcium, manganese, magnesium, and zinc. Choose a healthy store-bought sauce or make your own hoisin on page 173. Swap the soy sauce for tamari if you'd like it to be gluten-free.

SERVES 2

5 oz firm tofu
2-inch piece fresh ginger
2 garlic cloves
1 small fresh green chile
5 scallions
7 oz shiitake mushrooms
1 red bell pepper
1 medium carrot
3½ oz vegan noodles
   (we use whole wheat)
1 tbsp canola oil
½ tsp sesame oil
½ tsp maple syrup
½ tbsp hoisin sauce
2 tsp soy sauce
3½ oz bean sprouts
1 tsp sesame seeds
   (black/white/mixed)
salt and black pepper

TOFU PRESS OR 2 CLEAN TEA TOWELS AND A WEIGHT SUCH AS A HEAVY BOOK | VEGETABLE PEELER | BOILING WATER | WOK

First, prep your ingredients | Press the tofu using a tofu press or place it between two clean tea towels, lay it on a plate, and put a weight on top | Leave for 10 minutes to drain off any liquid and firm up | Peel the ginger by scraping off the skin with a spoon, then cut it into very fine matchsticks | Peel and thinly slice the garlic | Rip the stem from the chile, halve it lengthwise, remove the seeds, and slice thinly | Trim and thinly slice the scallions | Roughly chop the shiitake mushrooms | Trim, halve, core, and thinly slice the bell pepper | Peel the carrot then cut it lengthwise into ribbons using the vegetable peeler

Now, prep the noodles | Cook the noodles following the package instructions

Start making the stir-fry | Heat the canola oil in the wok over medium heat | Add the ginger, garlic, chile, and most of the scallions and cook, stirring, for 1 minute until fragrant | Add the sesame oil and maple syrup and stir for 30 seconds | Crumble the pressed tofu into the wok and let it sit for a minute so it browns, then stir for 2–3 minutes | Add the shiitake mushrooms, bell pepper, and hoisin sauce and stir for 2–3 minutes

Finish the process and serve | Add the carrot to the wok and cook for 1 minute | Add the drained noodles | Add the soy sauce and toss to combine | Cook, stirring, for 2 minutes | Add the bean sprouts and stir (or toss) for 1 minute | Toss and season to perfection with salt and pepper | Serve the noodles in bowls, garnished with the remaining scallions and the sesame seeds

628 KCAL | LOW FAT | LOW SUGAR | FULL OF FIBER | PROTEIN PACKED

PUTTANESCA POTATO STEW

This Miguel Barclay-inspired bowl uses new potatoes in place of pasta. The sauce is ready in minutes and is full of flavor—try it on pasta instead if you like, though. Olives, as well as adding little bites of extra taste, are also a good source of heart-healthy fats.

SERVES 4

- 1 lb 10 oz new potatoes
- 1 echalion (banana shallot)
- 3 garlic cloves
- 2 oz pitted Kalamata olives (or other black olives)
- 1 tsp olive oil
- ½ tsp fennel seeds
- ¼ tsp Italian seasoning
- ½ tsp chile flakes, plus extra to taste
- 1 tsp tomato paste
- 3 tbsp red wine
- 1⅔ cups canned tomato purée
- 4 oz fresh spinach leaves
- salt and black pepper
- 11 fresh basil leaves, to garnish

2 LARGE SAUCEPANS | FINE GRATER OR MICROPLANE

First, cook the potatoes | Wash the potatoes, halve any larger ones, then put them in one of the large saucepans with a pinch of salt | Cover with cold water, place over high heat, and bring to a rolling boil | Cook the potatoes for 12–15 minutes, until tender | Drain and set to one side

Now, start the puttanesca sauce | Peel and finely chop the shallot | Peel and grate the garlic cloves | Roughly chop the olives

Heat the olive oil in the second saucepan over medium heat | Add the shallot and a pinch of salt and stir for 1 minute | Add the garlic, fennel seeds, Italian seasoning, and chile flakes and cook, stirring, for 1 minute until aromatic | Add the tomato paste and stir for 30 seconds | Add the red wine, stir, and simmer for 3–4 minutes, until most of the liquid has evaporated

Add the tomato purée to the pan, stir through, and simmer for 7–8 minutes, until thickened | Add the new potatoes and fold them into the sauce | Add the spinach and stir until wilted | Add the olives | Taste the sauce, season to perfection with salt and pepper (and more chile if you like), and serve with a garnish of basil leaves

261 KCAL | LOW FAT | LOW SUGAR | FULL OF FIBER

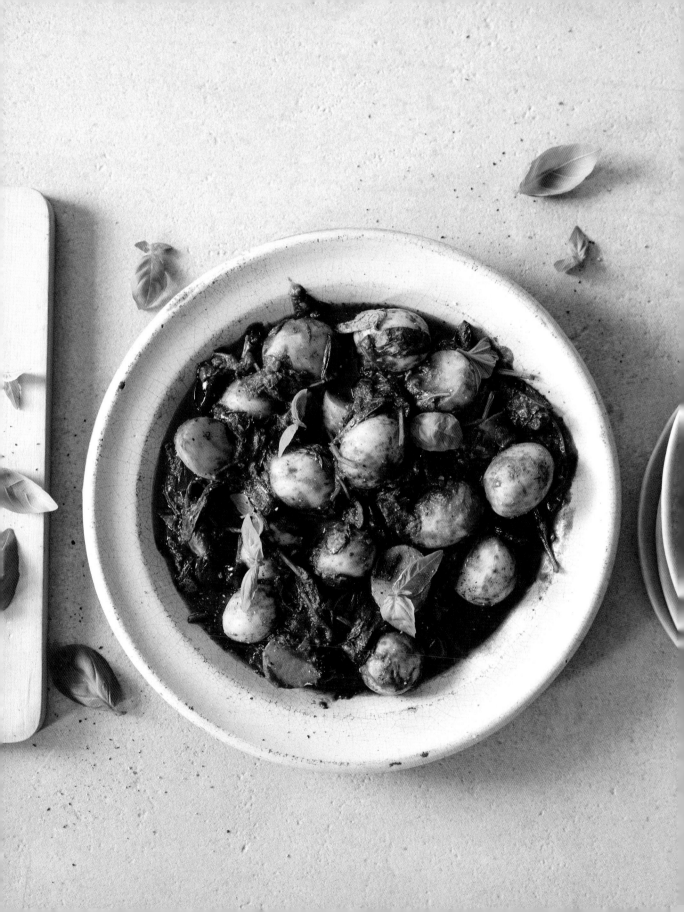

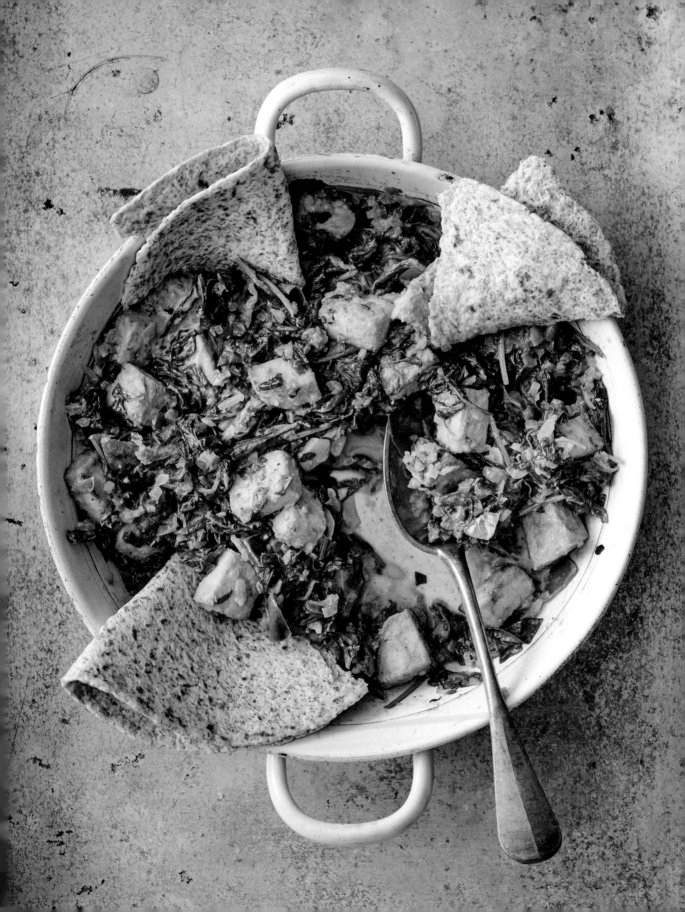

HEALTHY SAAG PANEER

We've re-created the mildly acidic taste and springy texture of paneer by flavoring tofu with a combination of nutritional yeast, miso, and lemon. Spinach is a great addition to a curry and you can pack in loads, as it wilts down so quickly. Go for whole wheat chapatis on the side.

SERVES 2

FOR THE TOFU PANEER

9 oz firm tofu
1 lemon
2 tbsp nutritional yeast
1 tbsp white miso paste
1 tsp coconut oil (melted)

FOR THE SAAG

1 onion
2 garlic cloves
2-inch piece fresh ginger (about ½ oz)
2 tomatoes
16 oz fresh spinach leaves
1 tbsp olive oil
1 tsp cumin seeds
2 tsp garam masala
½ tsp ground turmeric
½ tsp chile flakes
2 tbsp soy cream
salt and black pepper

TO SERVE

2 store-bought whole wheat chapatis or roti (or cooked brown rice)

PREHEAT OVEN TO 350°F | LINE A SHEET PAN WITH PARCHMENT PAPER | TOFU PRESS OR 2 CLEAN TEA TOWELS AND A WEIGHT SUCH AS A HEAVY BOOK | FINE GRATER OR MICROPLANE | LARGE SKILLET

First, make the paneer | Press the tofu using a tofu press or place it between two clean tea towels, lay it on a plate, and put a weight on top | Leave for at least 30 minutes to drain off any liquid and firm up | Zest, halve, and juice the lemon into a mixing bowl | Add the nutritional yeast, miso paste, and coconut oil and mix with a fork to combine | Cut the pressed tofu into ½-inch cubes | Tip the cubes into the mixing bowl, toss to coat, and leave to marinate for 25–30 minutes | Spread the cubes out on the lined sheet pan, put the pan in the oven, and bake for 20–30 minutes, until golden, turning them once, halfway through the cooking time

Now, make the saag | Peel and finely dice the onion | Peel and grate the garlic | Peel the ginger by scraping off the skin with a spoon, then grate it | Dice the tomatoes | Roughly chop the spinach

Heat the oil in the large skillet over medium heat | Add the cumin seeds and stir for 30 seconds | Add the onion and a pinch of salt and cook, stirring, for 5–7 minutes | Add the garlic and ginger and stir for 1 minute | Add the garam masala, turmeric, and chile flakes and stir for 30 seconds | Add the tomatoes and stir for 3–4 minutes | Add the spinach and stir for 2 minutes | Finally, add the soy cream and stir for 2 minutes, until the saag has a creamy consistency | Taste the saag and season to perfection with salt and pepper

Transfer the saag to a serving bowl | Take the paneer out of the oven | Place the paneer cubes on the saag and serve immediately with brown rice, whole wheat chapatis, or roti

716 KCAL | LOW SUGAR | FULL OF FIBER | PROTEIN PACKED

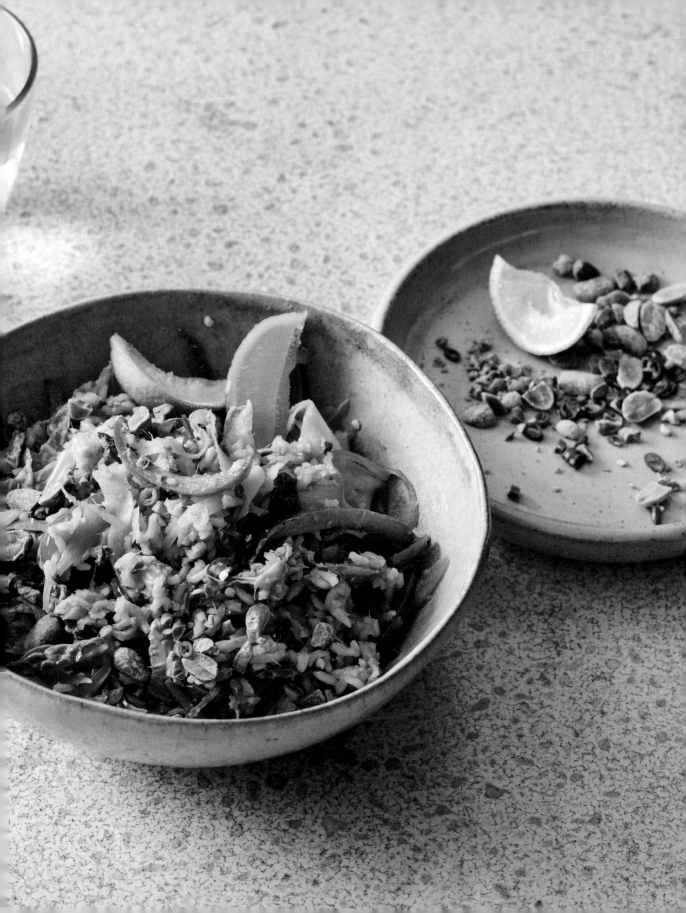

NASI GORENG

A classic fried rice dish from Indonesia, this meat-free version has all the delicious traditional umaminess from the added tomato paste, maple syrup, peanuts, and soy sauce.

SERVES 2

FOR THE SPICE PASTE

2 echalions (banana shallots)

1 lemongrass stalk

2-inch piece fresh ginger

2 garlic cloves

2 bird's-eye chiles

2 tbsp water

1 tsp tomato paste

1 tsp maple syrup

½ tsp sesame oil

2 oz unsalted roasted peanuts

1 lime

small handful of cilantro leaves

1 bird's-eye chile

2 echalions (banana shallots)

1 large carrot

1 red bell pepper

7 oz cabbage

1 tbsp olive oil

1 tbsp soy sauce

1 (8.5 oz) bag microwavable brown basmati rice

salt and black pepper

First, make the spice paste | Peel and roughly chop the shallots | Remove the tough outer layer of the lemongrass stalk and roughly chop the tender inner layers | Peel the ginger by scraping off the skin with a spoon, then roughly chop | Peel and roughly chop the garlic | Trim the chiles | Put all the paste ingredients in the blender and blitz to a paste

Roughly chop the peanuts | Cut the lime into wedges | Roughly chop the cilantro | Rip the stem from the chile, thinly slice, and set aside

Now, prep the vegetables | Peel and thinly slice the shallots lengthwise | Peel the carrot, then cut it lengthwise into long ribbons using the vegetable peeler | Trim, halve, core, and cut the bell pepper into strips | Halve, core and finely shred the cabbage

Cook the nasi goreng | Heat the olive oil in the wok or large skillet over high heat | Add the shallots and fry for 2–3 minutes, stirring regularly until softened | Add the carrot and bell pepper and stir for another 2–3 minutes | Add the cabbage and soy sauce and stir for another 2–3 minutes | Tip the stir-fried vegetables onto a plate and set to one side | Return the wok to the heat, add the spice paste, and stir for 2 minutes, until very fragrant, loosening it with a little water if necessary

Add the cooked rice to the pan and fold it into the paste | Return the cooked vegetables to the pan and fold them into the rice until the rice and vegetables are warmed through | Taste and season to perfection with salt and pepper

Plate up the nasi goreng, sprinkle over the peanuts, cilantro, and chile, and serve with a wedge of lime

485 KCAL | LOW SUGAR | FULL OF FIBER | PROTEIN PACKED

KEEMA ALOO

This Pakistani dish delivers a whopping amount of protein—just make sure you choose high-quality, low-saturated-fat vegan crumbles. For a curry feast to share, try serving it alongside our Saag Paneer on page 73 and some whole wheat chapatis.

SERVES 4

1 lb new potatoes
1 large onion
3 garlic cloves
2-inch piece fresh ginger (about ¾ oz)
1 fresh green chile
20 sprigs fresh cilantro
4 tsp ground turmeric
2 tbsp vegetable oil
2 tsp garam masala
1 tsp ground cumin
14 oz vegan crambles
1 (14.5 oz) can diced tomatoes
1½ cups frozen peas
salt and black pepper

TO SERVE

1 fresh green chile
1 scallion
4 whole wheat chapatis

FINE GRATER OR MICROPLANE | LARGE SAUCEPAN | LARGE, DEEP SKILLET

Wash the potatoes and cut them into equal bite-sized chunks | Peel and finely dice the onion | Peel and grate the garlic | Peel the ginger by scraping off the skin with a spoon, then grate it | Rip the stem from the chile, remove the seeds (if you prefer a milder curry), and thinly slice | Pick the cilantro leaves and finely chop the stems

Put the potatoes in the large saucepan and cover with cold water | Add a generous pinch of salt and 2 teaspoons of the turmeric | Put the pan over high heat and bring to a boil | When the water hits a rolling boil, cook the potatoes for 10–12 minutes, until tender | Drain the potatoes in a colander and let them steam-dry

Warm the oil in the large, deep skillet over medium heat | Add the onion and a small pinch of salt and cook, stirring, for 5–6 minutes | Add the garlic, ginger, cilantro stems and chile and cook, stirring, for another 2 minutes | Add the garam masala, cumin, and remaining turmeric and stir for 30 seconds | Add the vegan crumbles and cook for 6 minutes | Add the tomatoes and cook over low heat for 10 minutes | Add the peas and potatoes and stir gently for 2–3 minutes, until the peas have completely thawed | Add half the cilantro leaves and fold them into the keema for 30 seconds | Taste the keema and season to perfection with salt, pepper, and more garam masala

Spoon the keema aloo into bowls | Garnish with the remaining cilantro leaves, and some sliced green chile and scallion | Serve immediately with whole wheat chapatis

668 KCAL | LOW SUGAR | FULL OF FIBER | PROTEIN PACKED

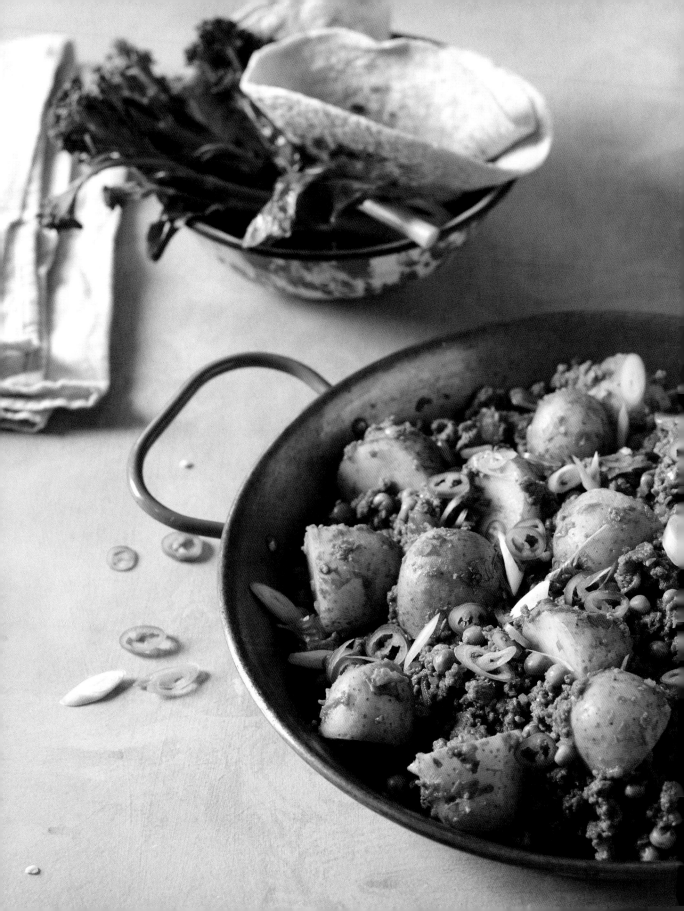

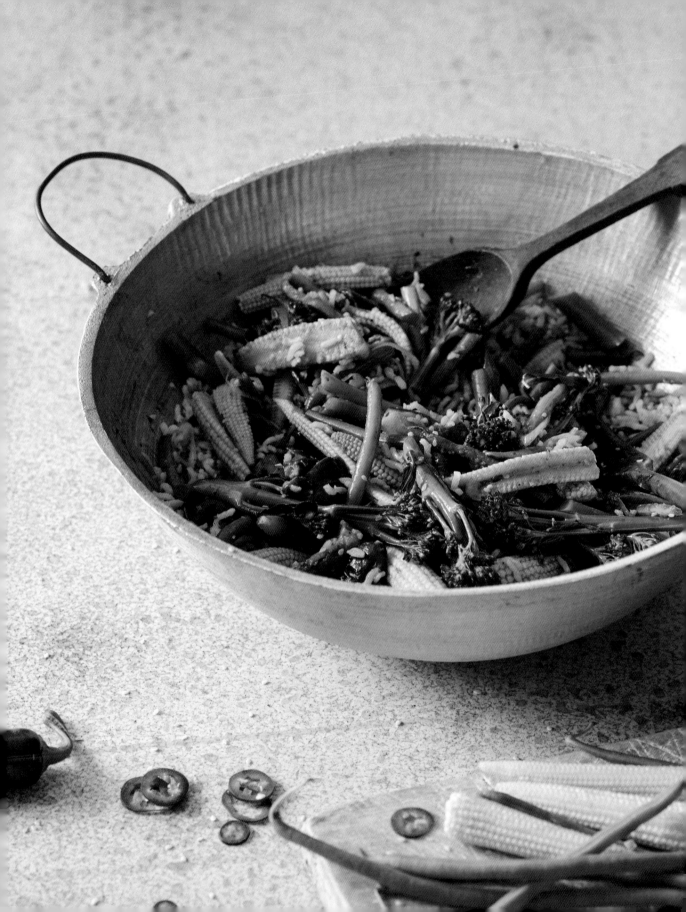

SPICY SICHUAN-STYLE SHIITAKE STIR-FRY

Stir-fries are a wonderful way to get loads of fresh, colorful veggies onto your plate. Our stir-fry rule is cook 'em hot and keep 'em crunchy! Shiitake mushrooms are high in vitamin B5, which the body needs to process fats and carbohydrates. The sauce is really moreish, packed with umami and spice.

SERVES 4

FOR THE SICHUAN-STYLE SAUCE

2 tbsp maple syrup
2 tbsp soy sauce
1 tbsp sriracha
1½ tbsp rice vinegar
½ tsp Chinese five-spice
1 tsp chile flakes

10 oz shiitake mushrooms
7 oz green beans
3½ oz baby corn
3½ oz broccolini
1-inch piece fresh ginger
1 garlic clove
2 scallions
1 fresh red chile
2 tsp vegetable oil
1 tsp sesame oil
2 (8.8 oz) bags microwavable brown basmati rice
2 tbsp white sesame seeds

FINE GRATER OR MICROPLANE | WOK | SAUCEPAN

First, make the Sichuan-style sauce | Put the maple syrup, soy sauce, sriracha, rice vinegar, Chinese five-spice, and chile flakes in a bowl and stir to combine

Now, prep the vegetables | Roughly chop the shiitake mushrooms | Trim and halve the green beans | Halve the baby corn lengthwise | Trim off and discard the tough ends of the broccolini and cut each broccoli stalk into thirds | Peel the ginger by scraping off the skin with a spoon, then finely grate | Peel and finely grate the garlic | Trim and thinly slice the scallions | Rip the stem from the chile and thinly slice

Heat the vegetable oil in the wok over medium heat | Add the ginger and garlic and stir for 30 seconds until aromatic | Add the shiitake mushrooms and stir-fry for 1 minute | Add half the sauce and stir for 1 minute | Add the green beans and stir for 3 minutes | Add the corn and broccoli | Add the remaining sauce and stir for another minute until the vegetables are cooked, but still have some bite | If the sauce needs loosening, add a splash of water, stir, and turn the heat right down | Drizzle over the sesame oil and toss together to combine

Cook the rice according to the package instructions | Once cooked, add half the sliced scallions to the rice | Put the rice in bowls and add the stir-fry | Garnish with the remaining scallions and the sliced chile, sprinkle over the sesame seeds, and serve Immediately

387 KCAL | LOW SUGAR | FULL OF FIBER | PROTEIN PACKED

TOM YUMMO SOUP

A long-time favorite of Henry's, this is his version of tom yum soup. There are so many layers of flavor that every single spoonful is a taste sensation! Using light coconut milk helps keep it lower in saturated fat, and yet it's still creamy and delicious.

SERVES 4

2 lemongrass stalks
2 red onions
7 oz button mushrooms
1 tbsp plus
    1 tsp vegetable oil
2 cups vegetable stock
3 cups water
generous ¾ cup reduced-fat coconut milk
1 tbsp soy sauce
4 tsp maple syrup

FOR THE PASTE

2½-inch piece fresh ginger
6 garlic cloves
2 fresh red Thai chiles
7 oz cherry tomatoes
40 sprigs fresh cilantro (about 1½ oz)
1 lime
scant 3 tbsp vegan Thai red curry paste
4 tsp tomato paste

TO SERVE

1 lime
4 scallions

BLENDER | SOUP POT

First, prep the ingredients | Peel away and discard the hard outer bark of the lemongrass and thinly slice the tender stalk | Peel and slice the onions | Quarter the mushrooms | Peel the ginger by scraping off the skin with a spoon | Peel the garlic | Rip the stems from the Thai chiles, cut them in half lengthwise and remove the seeds if you prefer, then roughly chop | Halve the cherry tomatoes | Pick the cilantro leaves and roughly chop the stems | Juice the lime | Quarter the lime for serving, and trim and slice the scallions into strips lengthwise

Now, make the paste | Put the ginger, garlic, chiles, cherry tomatoes, cilantro stems, lime juice, red curry paste, and tomato paste in the blender and blitz to a paste

Time to make your soup | Heat the vegetable oil in the soup pot over medium-high heat | Add the lemongrass and onion and cook, stirring, for 5–7 minutes | Add the mushrooms and stir for 5–7 minutes, until they have softened and any water that has come out of the mushrooms has evaporated | Add the curry paste and stir for 3–4 minutes, until fragrant | Add the stock, water, coconut milk, soy sauce, and maple syrup, stir, bring to a boil, reduce the heat, and simmer gently for 30–40 minutes

When the soup is thick and rich, taste it and adjust the seasoning accordingly, adding lime juice, soy sauce, or pepper as needed | Ladle the soup into bowls and serve immediately, garnished with scallion and cilantro and the lime quarters for squeezing

238 KCAL | LOW FAT | LOW SUGAR | FULL OF FIBER

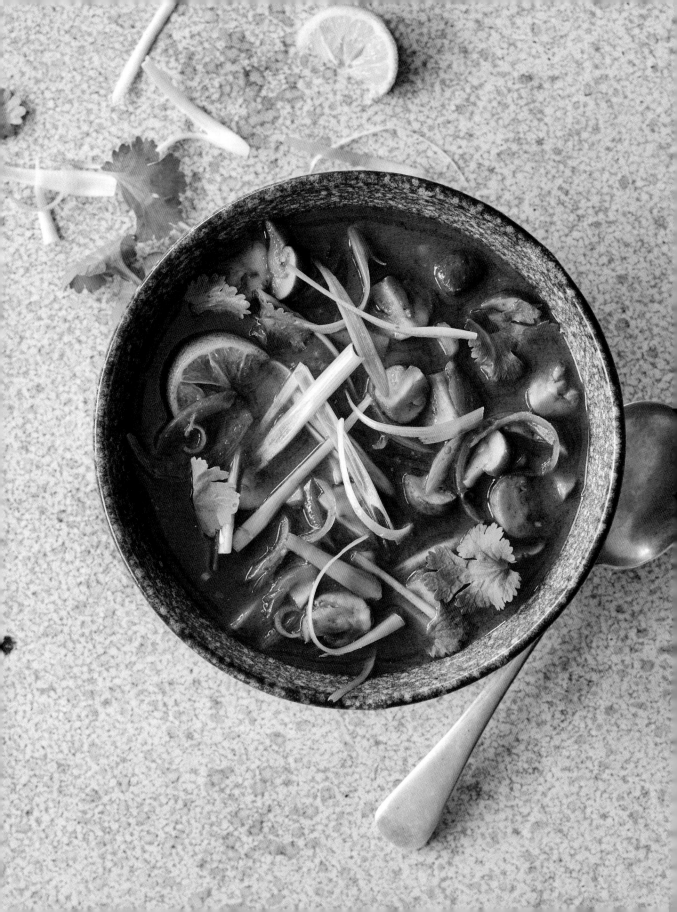

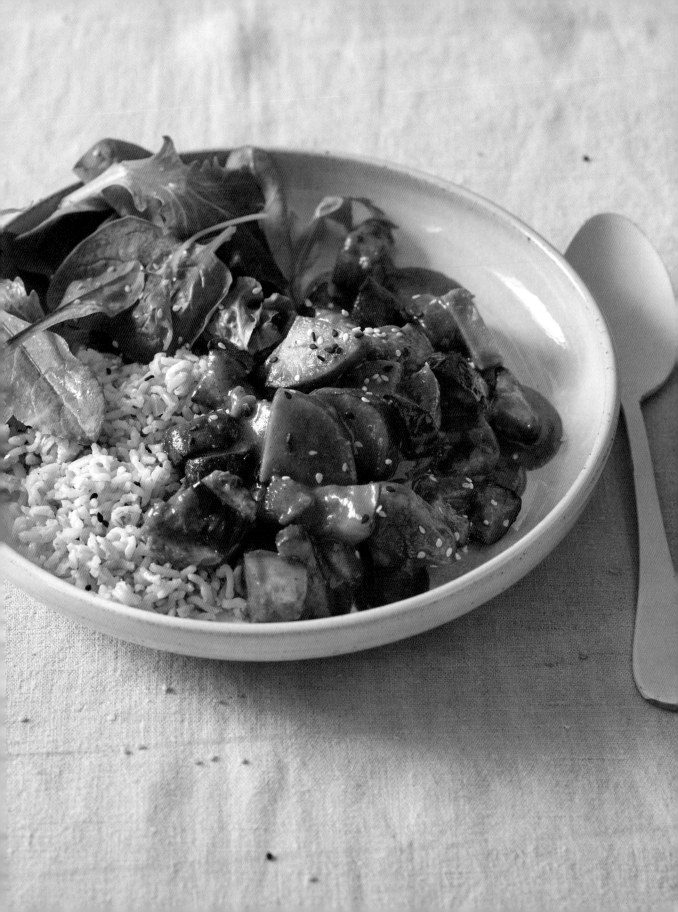

MIXED VEG KATSU CURRY

Roasting veg in the oven first is an easy way of adding extra flavor. The curry sauce is light and fresh tasting, and it's amazing with any veg you might have at home, so feel free to play around with the ingredients. This quick meal will give you a real nutritional boost thanks to the miso, sweet potato, eggplant, zucchini, and mixed greens.

SERVES 4

FOR THE ROAST VEGETABLES

1 large sweet potato (about 12 oz)
1 large eggplant
1 large zucchini
2 garlic cloves
½ tbsp olive oil
1 tbsp white miso paste

FOR THE KATSU SAUCE

1 onion
2 garlic cloves
½ tbsp olive oil
a pinch of salt
1 tbsp soy sauce
2 tbsp curry powder
2 tsp maple syrup
½ tsp ground turmeric
½ tsp sambar (or garam masala)
⅔ cup reduced-fat coconut milk
1 cup vegetable stock

TO SERVE

4 cups cooked basmati rice or 2 (8.8 oz) bags microwaveable brown basmati rice
3½ oz mixed salad greens
1 tbsp sesame seeds (black/white/mixed)

PREHEAT OVEN TO 400°F | LINE A SHEET PAN WITH PARCHMENT PAPER | FINE GRATER OR MICROPLANE | DEEP SKILLET | FOOD PROCESSOR

First, prep the roast vegetables | Wash, trim, and cut the sweet potato and eggplant into ½-inch chunks | Trim the zucchini, halve lengthwise, then cut into ½-inch sices | Peel and grate the garlic

Put the olive oil and garlic in a large bowl, add the white miso paste and a splash of water, and stir to form a thick paste | Add the sweet potato, eggplant, and zucchini and toss so they are well coated in the paste

Use tongs to transfer the sweet potato and eggplant pieces to |the lined sheet pan, put the pan in the oven, and roast for 10 minutes | Take the pan out of the oven, add the zucchinis, put the pan back into the oven, and roast for another 20 minutes

While the vegetables are roasting, make the katsu sauce | Peel and finely dice the white onion | Peel and grate the garlic

Heat the olive oil in the deep skillet over medium heat | Add the onion to the pan with the salt and cook, stirring, for 10 minutes, until soft | Add the garlic and stir for 1 minute | Reduce the heat slightly, add the soy sauce, curry powder, maple syrup, turmeric, and sambar and stir for 1 minute to combine | Add the coconut milk to the pan, stir to combine, increase the temperature, and bring the sauce to a gentle simmer | Add the stock, stir, bring back to a gentle simmer, and cook for about 10 minutes, until the sauce has darkened in color significantly | Transfer the sauce to the food processor and blitz until totally smooth | The sauce should be the consistency of double cream, so add a tablespoon or two of water to thin it down if necessary

Take the vegetables out of the oven, transfer them to the pan of sauce, and fold them in | Heat the rice, if necessary, or cook it following the package instructions | Plate up the rice, curry, and salad greens | Sprinkle with the sesame seeds and serve immediately

320 KCAL | LOW FAT | LOW SUGAR | FULL OF FIBER

CRISPY TOFU SATAY BITES

These high-protein bites are great for a post-workout snack—or for serving up at a party! Baking instead of deep-frying them helps keep everything lean, and makes the recipe easier, too. And the dipping sauce is incredible.

SERVES 4 AS A SNACK

PREHEAT OVEN TO 325°F | LINE A SHEET PAN WITH PARCHMENT PAPER | TOFU PRESS OR 2 CLEAN TEA TOWELS AND A WEIGHT SUCH AS A HEAVY BOOK | BLENDER

FOR THE TOFU NUGGETS

10 oz firm tofu
1 tbsp Thai 7-spice
½ tsp ground turmeric
½ tsp ground black pepper
1 tbsp plant-based yogurt
4 tbsp cornstarch
cooking oil spray
¼ cup cilantro leaves
salt

FOR THE SATAY DIPPING SAUCE

1 small garlic clove
1 lime
3 tbsp smooth peanut or almond butter
1 tbsp maple syrup
1 tsp soy sauce
½ tbsp vegan Thai red curry paste
¼ cup water

First, prep the tofu | Press the tofu using a tofu press or place it between two clean tea towels, lay it on a plate, and put a weight on top | Leave for 10–15 minutes to drain off any liquid | Carefully rip the tofu into equal bite-sized nuggets (the rough edges from ripping it aid crunchiness)

Put the tofu nuggets in a mixing bowl, add the Thai 7-spice, turmeric, and pepper, and season with a little salt | Gently toss to coat | Add the yogurt and fold to coat | Add 1 tablespoon of the cornstarch and fold again, to coat | Repeat this process twice more, adding a tablespoon of cornstarch at a time | Add the final tablespoon of cornstarch to the bowl and toss the nuggets to coat

Tip the nuggets onto the lined sheet pan and spread them out | Spray with 4 sprays of cooking oil, put the pan in the oven, and bake for 25 minutes, turning the nuggets halfway through to break them up (if the nuggets appear to be drying out too quickly, spray a touch more cooking spray over the top of them)

While the nuggets are baking, make the satay dipping sauce | Peel the garlic clove | Halve the lime and squeeze the juice into a blender | Add all the remaining sauce ingredients and blitz to make a creamy sauce

Time to serve! | Remove the nuggets from the oven, put them on a dish, and garnish with cilantro leaves | Put the satay dipping sauce in a serving bowl alongside and serve immediately

299 KCAL | LOW SUGAR | PROTEIN PACKED

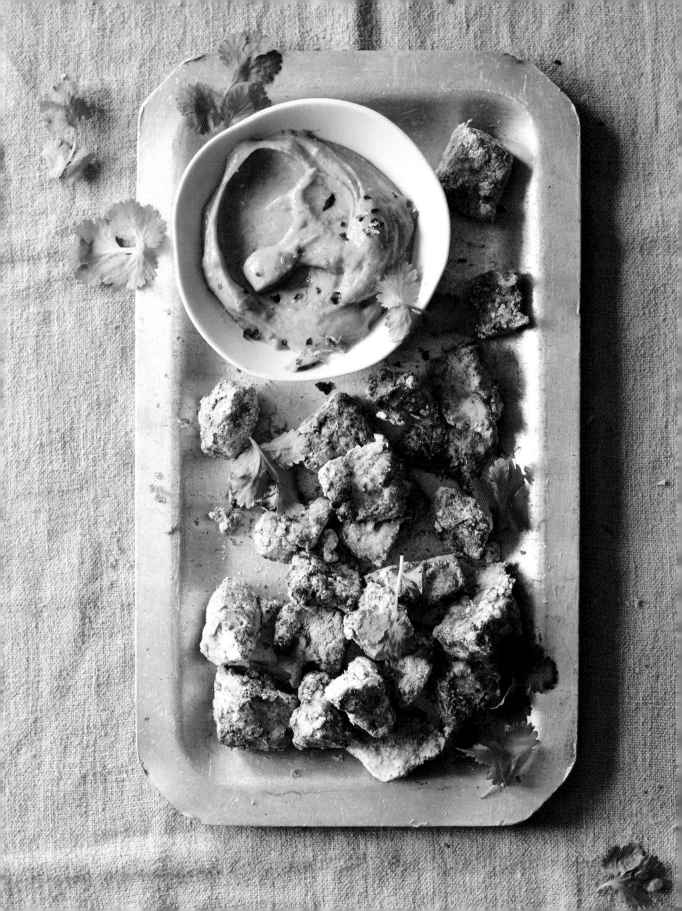

INDIAN SPICED TOMATO SOUP

A sweet, spicy, hearty bowl of soup is always welcome in the BOSH! household! While tomato soup is always great, tomato soup made with a loads of fresh tomatoes is about as good as it can get! Try it with a dollop of cooling plant-based yogurt and some crunchy whole wheat bread. You could also blend in some silken tofu for added protein and creaminess.

SERVES 4

2¼ lb cherry tomatoes

2 tsp extra-virgin olive oil, plus extra for drizzling

½ fresh red chile

2 garlic cloves

3 small green cardamom pods

½ tsp cumin seeds

1 tsp ground cilantro

½ tsp ground turmeric

½ tsp cayenne pepper

1 tsp ground black pepper

2 small red onions

1 tbsp balsamic vinegar

salt and black pepper

TO SERVE

fresh basil leaves, to garnish

4 slices whole wheat sourdough bread

PREHEAT OVEN TO 350°F | ROASTING PAN | 2 LARGE SAUCEPANS | BLENDER

Roast the tomatoes | Tip the tomatoes into the roasting pan | Drizzle over 1 teaspoon of the olive oil and season with salt and pepper | Cut the half chile lengthwise, remove the seeds, and add it to the pan | Crush the garlic cloves into the pan (skin on) | Crack open the cardamom pods and add the seeds to the pan | Cover the tomatoes with all the remaining spices | Mix everything around, put the pan in the oven, and roast for 15 minutes

Peel and finely chop the onions | Heat the remaining teaspoon of olive oil in one of the saucepans over medium heat | Add the onions and a pinch of salt and sauté for 8–10 minutes, stirring regularly | Add the balsamic vinegar and stir for 2 minutes

Remove the pan from the oven, removing the garlic skins, and put everything in the saucepan, making sure you scrape all the spices in | Stir the contents of the pan to combine | Pour half the contents of the pan into the blender and blitz until smooth (if you prefer a chunkier soup, blend only until roughly textured) | Pour the contents of the blender into a separate saucepan over low heat to keep warm, then blend the rest of the soup | Garnish with basil leaves, a drizzle of olive oil, and a sprinkle of salt and pepper, and serve with bread

384 KCAL | LOW FAT | LOW SUGAR | FULL OF FIBER | PROTEIN PACKED

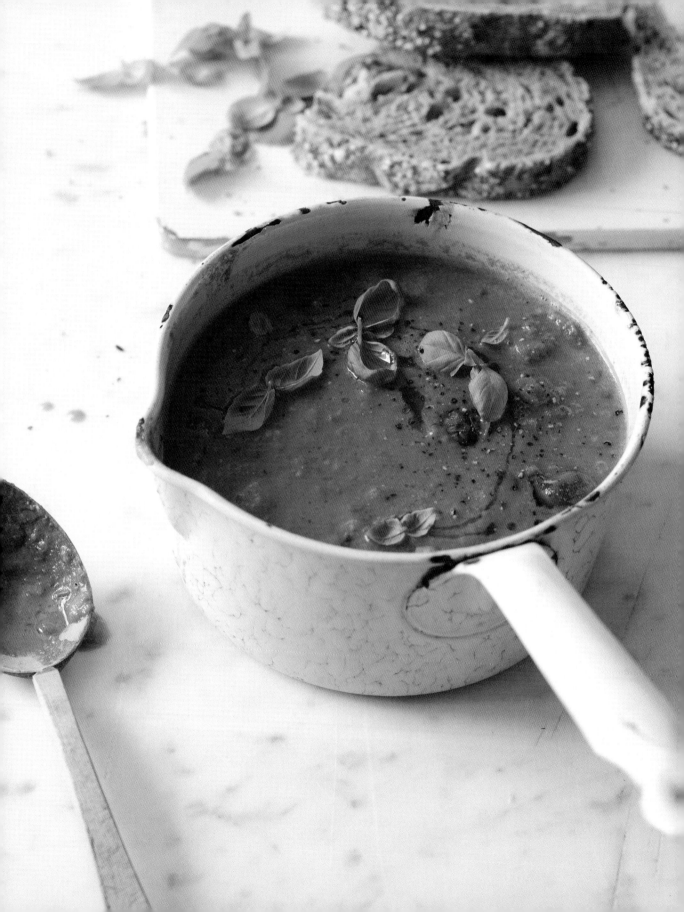

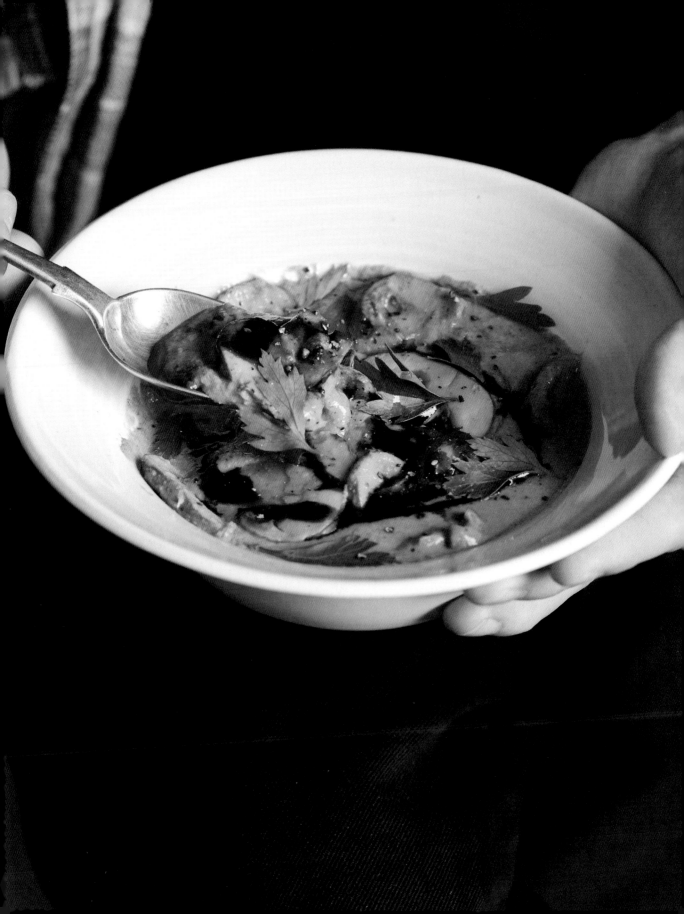

MUSHROOM SOUP

While messing about in the kitchen with our buddy Liam Chau, we created this lighter version of his favorite cream of mushroom soup. Use any mushrooms you like, but if you can, go for ones that are fortified with vitamin D. We add silken tofu for extra protein and creaminess.

SERVES 2

2 cups boiling water
½ oz dried mushrooms
3 echalions (banana shallots)
1 large garlic clove
14 oz fresh mushrooms
2 sprigs fresh rosemary
5 sprigs fresh thyme
1 tbsp olive oil
3 tbsp oat cream
5 oz silken tofu
salt and black pepper

TO SERVE

1 tsp extra-virgin olive oil
1 tsp balsamic vinegar
handful of fresh parsley
4 slices crusty
   whole wheat bread

BOILING WATER | 4-CUP GLASS MEASURING CUP | FINE GRATER OR MICROPLANE | SOUP POT | BLENDER

First, soak the mushrooms | Pour the boiling water into the measuring cup, add the dried mushrooms and a pinch of salt, stir to combine, and set aside for 5 minutes, until the water is a dark caramel color

While the mushrooms are soaking, prep the remaining ingredients | Peel and dice the shallots | Peel and grate the garlic | Cut the fresh mushrooms into scant ¼-inch-thick slices | Pick the rosemary and thyme leaves from the sprigs and finely chop

Now, start making the soup | Heat the olive oil in the soup pot over medium heat | Add the shallots and cook, stirring, for 3–4 minutes | Add the garlic and stir for 1 minute | Add the mushrooms, rosemary, and thyme and stir for 7–8 minutes, until the mushrooms are well cooked down

Add the mushroom stock to the soup, pouring it through a sieve into the pan, reserving the rehydrated dried mushrooms | Increase the heat and bring to a boil, stirring occasionally | Reduce the heat and pour in the cream while stirring

Finish the soup and serve | Transfer half the soup, the silken tofu, and the rehydrated dried mushrooms to the blender and blitz until smooth and thick | Pour the blended soup back into the pan, stir to combine, turn up the heat, and simmer for 2 minutes | Taste and season to perfection with salt and pepper | Ladle the soup into bowls, season with a grind of black pepper, and drizzle with the olive oil and balsamic vinegar | Pick the leaves from the parsley | Garnish with the parsley leaves and serve with whole wheat bread

418 KCAL | LOW FAT | LOW SUGAR | FULL OF FIBER | PROTEIN PACKED

SPICY LENTIL SOUP

High in protein, fiber, and flavor while being low in fat, this slightly fiery, warming soup is a perfect post-workout meal. Lentils are incredibly good for you as well as being tasty, and they add great texture to dishes; we try to eat them as often as we can.

SERVES 4

1 onion
3 carrots (about 12 oz)
generous ¾ cup red lentils
2 green cardamom pods
1 tbsp olive oil
4 scant tbsp tomato paste
½ tsp chile flakes,
    plus extra to taste
1 tsp smoked paprika
½ tsp ground cumin
½ tsp ground cilantro
1½ cups vegetable stock
4¼ cups hot water
5 oz kale
1 lime
1 tsp sumac
salt and black pepper

TO SERVE

4 tbsp plant-based yogurt
fresh cilantro leaves, for
    garnish
4 slices whole wheat
    bread

GRATER | PESTLE AND MORTAR | LARGE SOUP POT |
STICK BLENDER

Prep the vegetables | Peel and finely dice the onion | Peel and coarsely grate the carrots | Rinse the lentils

Put the cardamom pods in the mortar | Bash them with the pestle to release the seeds, then remove the pod skins and grind the seeds

Heat the olive oil in the soup pot over medium heat | Add the onion with a pinch of salt and cook, stirring, for 5–6 minutes until soft and translucent | Add the tomato paste, chile flakes, ground cardamom, smoked paprika, cumin, coriander, and 1 tsp black pepper and stir for 1 minute

Add the carrots and lentils and stir for 1 minute to combine and coat | Add the stock and hot water, stir, bring the heat up to a gentle simmer, and cook for 30–35 minutes, stirring regularly, until the lentils are cooked through and tender | Meanwhile, strip the midribs from the kale and thinly slice the leaves, and halve the lime

Add the sumac to the pan, add the juice of the lime, and stir it into the soup | Using a stick blender, blitz the soup until it reaches your desired level of smoothness | Add the kale, fold it into the soup, and simmer for another 3–4 minutes

Taste the soup and season to perfection with salt, pepper, and chile flakes | Serve in bowls, topped with yogurt and cilantro leaves, with whole wheat bread alongside

434 KCAL | LOW FAT | LOW SUGAR | FULL OF FIBER | PROTEIN PACKED

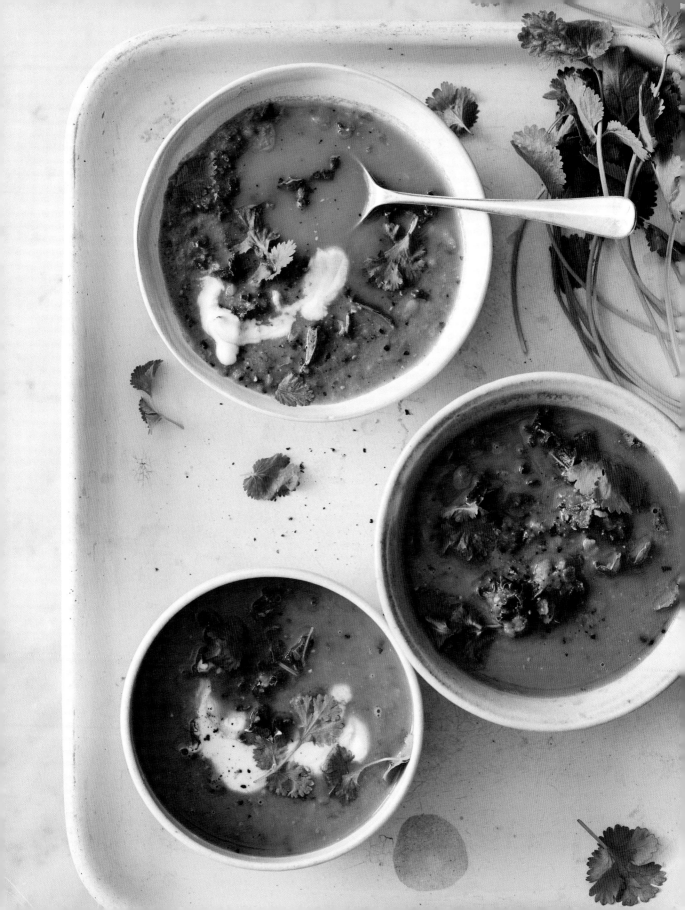

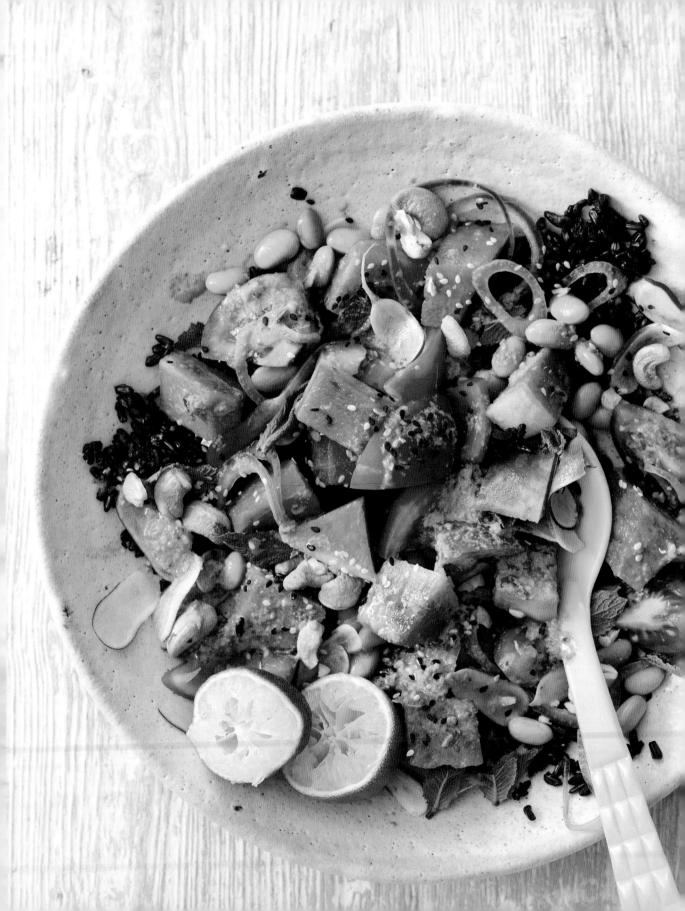

ZINGY WATERMELON SALAD

Our friend and all-round foodie whizz, Sophie Foot, gave us the inspiration for this delicious summer salad. Perfect for a balmy evening on the balcony, in the garden, or out of a Tupperware in the park! We love black rice as it's a great source of slow-burning fiber, while edamame are high in protein and folate, as well as adding an amazing color contrast.

SERVES 2

generous 1 cup black rice

generous ¾ cup frozen shelled edamame

1 lb watermelon

7 oz tomatoes

2 radishes

3 tbsp fresh mint leaves

1 oz unsalted cashews

1 tsp mix of black and white sesame seeds

FOR THE PICKLED ONION

1 red onion

1 tsp salt

1 tsp superfine sugar

⅔ cup apple cider vinegar

½ tsp whole black peppercorns

½ tsp fennel seeds

½ tsp cilantro seeds

1 bay leaf

FOR THE DRESSING

2 limes

1 small fresh red chile

1 small garlic clove

2-inch piece fresh ginger

1 tbsp sesame oil

1½ tsp mirin

1 tsp maple syrup

1 tsp soy sauce

SMALL SAUCEPAN | BOILING WATER | AIRTIGHT JAR | FINE GRATER OR MICROPLANE | SALAD BOWL

First, cook the rice and edamame following the package instructions

Now, make the pickled onion | Peel and thinly slice the onion | Put the salt, sugar, cider vinegar, peppercorns, fennel seeds, cilantro seeds, and bay leaf in the small saucepan and warm over a gentle heat until fragrant | Take the pan off the heat | Put the onion in a heatproof bowl, cover with boiling water, and leave to sit for 1 minute | Remove the onion from the bowl with a fork and transfer to the airtight jar | Pour the pickling liquid into the jar and seal | Once the jar is at room temperature, transfer it to the fridge | The pickle will keep for up to 1 month

Now, make the dressing | Juice the limes | Rip the stem from the chile, halve, remove the seeds, and finely chop | Peel and finely chop the garlic | Peel the ginger by scraping off the skin with a spoon, then grate | Put the lime juice, chile, garlic, ginger, sesame oil, mirin, maple syrup, and soy sauce in a bowl and mix | Add a splash of water to loosen, if necessary

Now, prep the salad | Cut the watermelon and tomatoes into bite-sized chunks | Trim and thinly slice the radishes | Tip the watermelon, tomatoes, radishes, and edamame into the salad bowl and gently toss to combine | Roughly tear the mint leaves | Add 2 tablespoons of the pickled onion (drained) and 1 tablespoon of the dressing and gently toss to combine

Now, assemble the salad | Layer the black rice on a plate, with a little dressing, then top with the watermelon, tomato, and onion mix | Lightly fold in the mint | Top with the cashews, sprinkle with the sesame seeds, and serve, with the rest of the dressing alongside

648 KCAL | LOW FAT

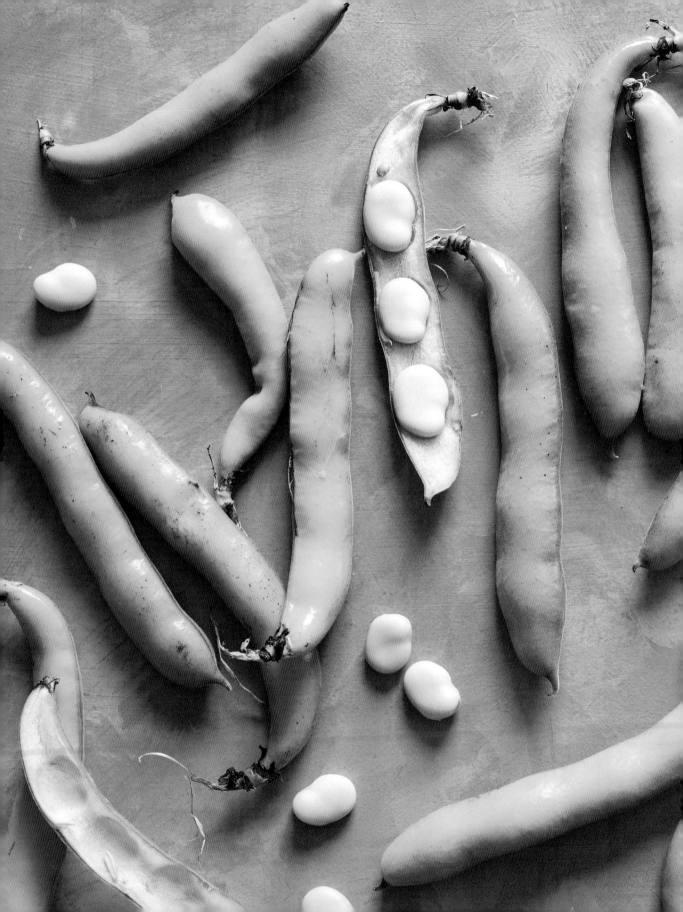

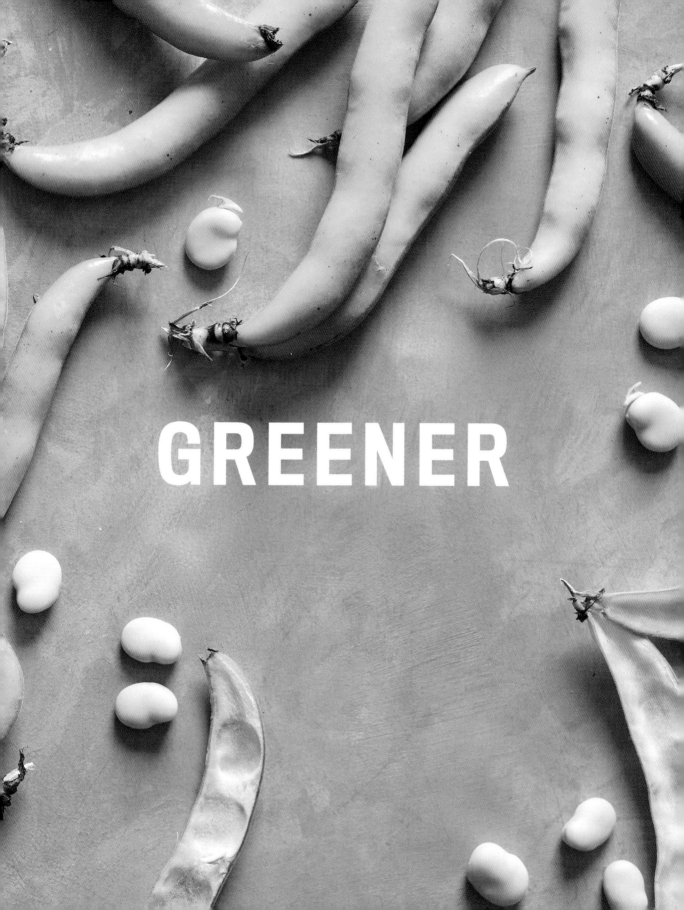

GREENER

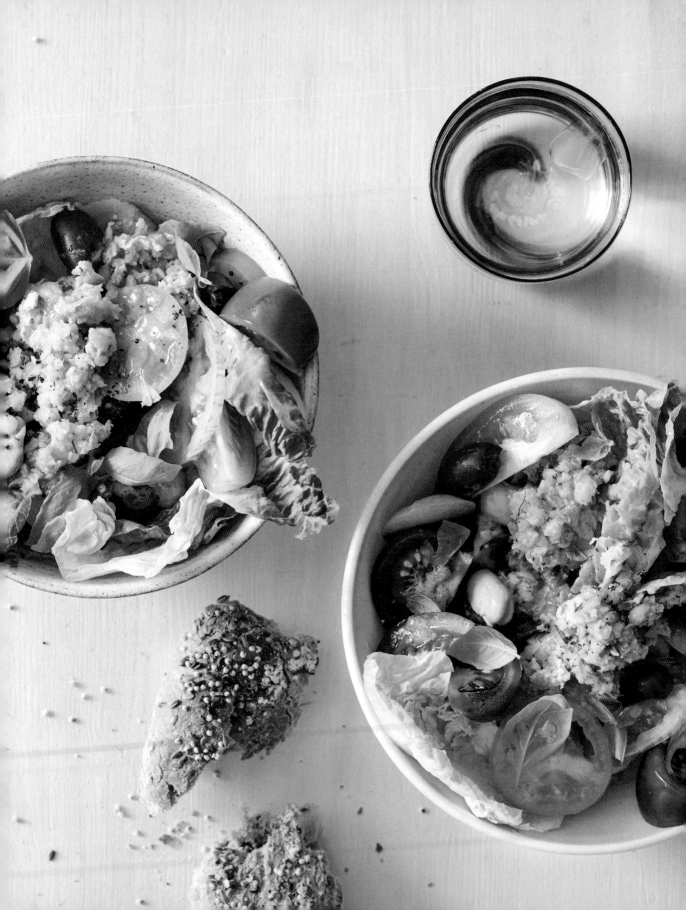

NIÇOISE SALAD

A tuna Niçoise salad used to be one of our favorite meals—fresh, protein-packed, and zingy with flavors of the sea. Here we've made a healthy, delicious, plant-based alternative, which still has all those great seaside flavors. If you want to make it even fishier, try adding one teaspoon of dulse flakes to the chickpea "tuna" mix.

SERVES 2

FINE GRATER OR MICROPLANE | POTATO MASHER

FOR THE CHICKPEA "TUNA"

1 (14 oz) can chickpeas
1 celery stalk
1 shallot
1 small carrot
2 small cornichons (or 4 capers)
1 lemon
1 sprig fresh dill
handful of fresh parsley
2 tbsp hummus
salt and black pepper

FOR THE DRESSING

1 small garlic clove
1 oz fresh basil sprigs
1 tbsp extra-virgin olive oil
1 tbsp white wine vinegar
1 tsp Dijon mustard

FOR THE SALAD

10 oz mixed tomatoes
2 Little Gem lettuces
5 oz shelled fava beans
1 oz pitted Kalamata (or other black) olives
crusty whole wheat bread, to serve, optional

First, make the "tuna" | Drain and rinse the chickpeas | Trim and very finely chop the celery | Peel and very finely chop the shallot | Peel and finely grate the carrot | Finely chop the cornichons | Zest and juice the lemon | Pick the dill and parsley leaves and finely chop

Mash the chickpeas in a bowl with a potato masher until they are crushed but still retain some texture | Add the celery, shallot, carrot, cornichons, lemon juice and zest, dill, parsley, and hummus to the bowl | Mix well and season to taste with salt and pepper

Now, make the dressing | Peel and grate the garlic | Pick the leaves from the basil stems and finely chop half the stems | In a mixing bowl, whisk the oil, vinegar, and mustard | Add the chopped basil stems to the dressing with the grated garlic (keep the basil leaves for the salad)

Now, make and assemble the salad | Quarter the tomatoes | Separate the lettuce leaves | Place the tomatoes, basil leaves, lettuce leaves, fava beans, and olives in the bowl of dressing and gently toss | Divide between two plates, top with the chickpea "tuna," and serve with crusty whole wheat bread (if using)

428 KCAL | LOW SUGAR | FULL OF FIBER | PROTEIN PACKED

BOSH! BURNT EGGPLANT

This is a gorgeous and fancy-looking dish that is definitely Instagram-worthy. All the fresh herbs, aromatics, and the miso dressing mean it's high in healthy flavor and the eggplant is hearty and filling. This works great as a main meal for two or a starter for four.

SERVES 2

2 eggplants
2 scallions
1 fresh long red chile
small handful of
   cilantro leaves
small handful of
   mint leaves
1 tsp white sesame seeds

FOR THE DRESSING

generous 1 tbsp white
   miso paste
¼ cup rice vinegar
1 tbsp maple syrup
1 tsp soy sauce
1 tsp tahini
2 tsp sesame oil
½ lime
salt and black pepper

PREHEAT BROILER TO HIGH | LINE A SHEET PAN WITH FOIL |
PASTRY BRUSH

First, prep the eggplant | Trim and cut the eggplant into ⅓-inch-thick slices with a very sharp knife and lay the slices on the lined sheet pan (you might have to broil them in batches) | Broil the eggplant for 3–4 minutes on each side, until almost completely softened–keep an eye on them as broiler temperatures will vary | They should be soft to the touch and slightly browned

Meanwhile, make the dressing and prep the garnish | Put the miso paste, rice vinegar, maple syrup, soy sauce, tahini, and sesame oil in a small mixing bowl | Squeeze in the lime juice and mix to combine | Taste and season to perfection with salt and pepper | Trim and thinly slice the scallions | Rip the stem from the chile and thinly slice

Once the eggplant has been pre-broiled, liberally brush dressing over the eggplant slices, keeping back about a quarter of the dressing for later | Put the pan back under the hot broiler and broil the eggplant for 4–5 minutes, until the slices are golden and completely soft

Time to plate up! | Plate up the eggplant slices and drizzle over any remaining dressing | Garnish the eggplant with the scallions, chile, cilantro, mint, and sesame seeds, and serve

226 KCAL | LOW FAT | LOW SUGAR | FULL OF FIBER | PROTEIN PACKED

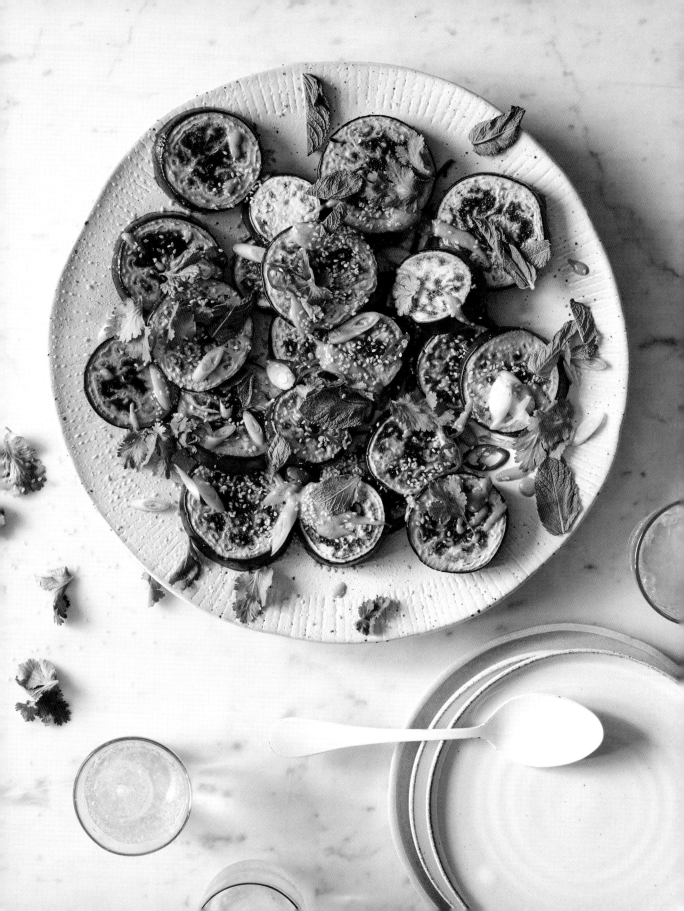

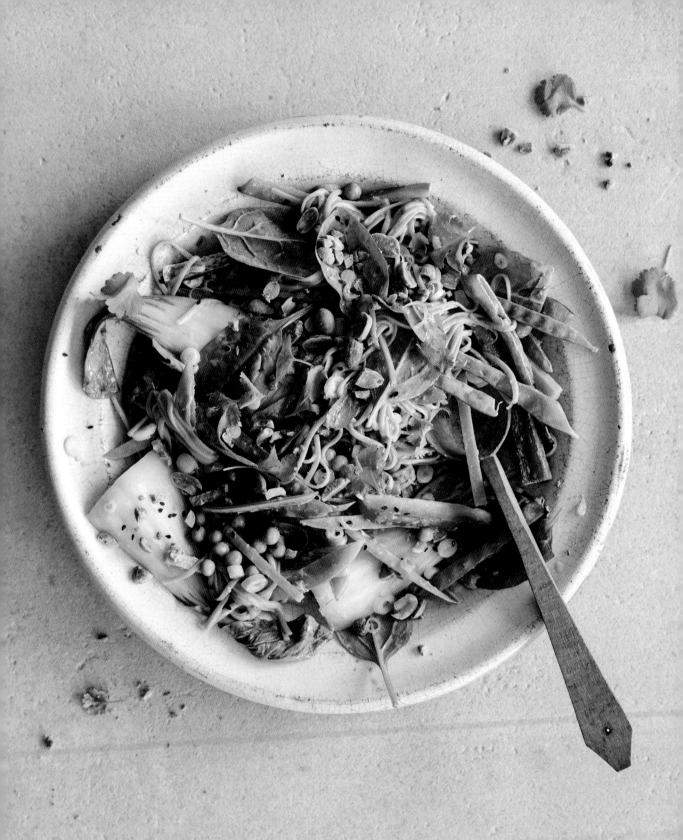

SATAY SALAD

We absolutely love the sweet, sour, peanutty flavors in a satay sauce, which we have used as a dressing in this easy salad. Packed with health-giving plants, this salad is a source of fiber and protein, and the addition of ginger is great for your digestive system.

SERVES 2

FOR THE SAUCE

1 large garlic clove
2-inch piece fresh ginger
1 lime
1 tbsp sesame oil
½ tsp chile flakes
4 tsp soy sauce
2 tsp maple syrup
4 tbsp smooth peanut butter
6 tbsp water

3½ oz soba noodles
¾ cup frozen peas
5 oz sugar snap peas or snow peas
2 heads bok choy
4 scallions
30 sprigs fresh cilantro
2 tbsp unsalted peanuts
1 lime
1 red bell pepper
1 medium carrot
1½ cups baby spinach
1 tbsp black sesame seeds

FINE GRATER OR MICROPLANE | SMALL SAUCEPAN | BOILING WATER | SALAD BOWL

First, make the sauce | Peel and grate the garlic | Peel the ginger by scraping off the skin with a spoon, then grate | Halve the lime | Heat the sesame oil over medium heat in the small saucepan | Add the garlic, ginger, and chile flakes and stir for 30 seconds, until aromatic | Reduce the heat to low, add the soy sauce and maple syrup, and stir to combine | Add the peanut butter and stir until well combined | Squeeze in the lime juice and stir | Add the water and stir until you have a smooth, creamy sauce | Take the pan off the heat and set to one side

Now, prep the noodles and veg | Cook the noodles following the package instructions | Put the peas in a heatproof bowl, cover with boiling water, and leave for 1 minute, then drain, reserving the water | Halve the sugar snap peas or snow peas lengthwise | Trim the bottom from the bok choy and add them to the pea water, setting aside the few middle (yellowish color) leaves first | Trim the scallions, thinly slice half of them, and cut the rest into strips lengthwise | Pick the cilantro leaves | Lightly crush the peanuts | Cut the lime into wedges | Trim, halve, core, and slice the bell pepper | Peel and cut the carrot into thin strips | Drain the water from the peas and bok choy and rinse in a colander or sieve under the cold tap to cool

Now, build the salad | Add the noodles to a salad bowl and stir in the sauce, coating completely | Add the peas, sugar snap peas or snow peas, bok choy, thinly sliced scallions, bell pepper, carrot, and spinach to the bowl and toss to combine, making sure everything is well mixed | Serve the salad in two bowls, sprinkle over the remaining scallions, cilantro, black sesame seeds, and peanuts | Squeeze over lime wedges and serve immediately

714 KCAL | LOW SUGAR | FULL OF FIBER | PROTEIN PACKED

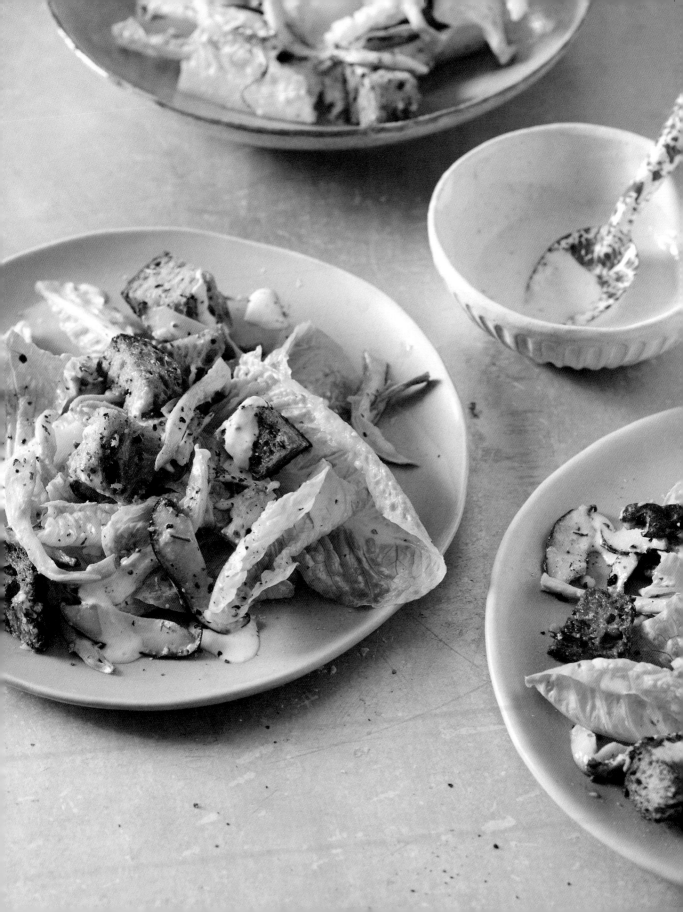

CAESAR SALAD

Chicken Caesar salad is such a classic dish. It was apparently invented in Mexico by a restaurant owner, aiming to bring Americans to his establishment. Either way, it's definitely a crowd-pleaser! We have reinvented it here using mushrooms and nutritional yeast, both of which are packed full of healthy vitamins and nutrients.

SERVES 4

FOR THE "CHICKEN"

9 king oyster mushrooms

1 tbsp olive oil

2 tbsp vegan-friendly chicken seasoning

FOR THE CROUTONS

7 oz unsliced seeded brown bread

2 tsp olive oil

1 tsp Italian seasoning

½ tsp garlic powder

FOR THE DRESSING

1 garlic clove

2 tbsp nutritional yeast

4 tbsp vegan mayonnaise

1 tbsp white wine vinegar

½ lemon

10 oz romaine lettuce

salt and black pepper

1 tbsp nutritional yeast, to serve, optional

PREHEAT OVEN TO 350°F | LINE A ROASTING PAN WITH PARCHMENT PAPER | LINE A SHEET PAN WITH PARCHMENT PAPER | FINE GRATER OR MICROPLANE

First, prep the "chicken" | Cut the caps off the king oyster mushrooms and slice them thinly | Pull the prongs of two forks along the length of the mushroom stems, roughly tearing them into matchsticks 1–2 inches long | Put the mushrooms in a bowl, drizzle with the olive oil, and sprinkle over the chicken seasoning | Toss to combine, making sure the mushrooms are evenly coated with the flavoring | Add the mushrooms to the roasting pan and make sure they are evenly spaced out | Put the pan in the oven, and bake the mushrooms for 25–30 minutes

Now, make the croutons | Cut the bread into 1-inch cubes | Put the olive oil, Italian seasoning, garlic powder, and a pinch each of salt and pepper in a bowl and stir to combine | Add the bread cubes and toss to combine, making sure the cubes are well coated | Spread the cubes out on the lined sheet pan, put the pan in the oven, and bake for 15 minutes, until golden and crispy

Make the salad dressing | Peel and grate the garlic clove | Put the garlic, nutritional yeast, vegan mayonnaise, and white wine vinegar in a mixing bowl | Grate the lemon zest into the bowl, squeeze in the juice, and stir to combine | Taste the dressing and season to perfection with salt and pepper | Add a splash of water if the dressing needs loosening

Assemble the salad | Trim and roughly chop the lettuce | Add the lettuce, the pulled and sliced oyster mushrooms, and half the croutons to a serving bowl and toss to combine | Sprinkle the remaining croutons over the salad, and the tablespoon of nutritional yeast (if using), drizzle with dressing, and serve immediately

372 KCAL | LOW SUGAR | FULL OF FIBER | PROTEIN PACKED

MIDDLE EASTERN SPICED CHICKPEA SALAD

A gorgeous rainbow of a salad, this one pops with red, orange, green, and a creamy, sesame-colored dressing. The chickpeas are coated with flavorful spices and roasted to add an extra nutty crunch. This dish is a great source of fiber and protein and will leave you feeling like you've really done yourself some good.

SERVES 4

FOR THE SPICED CHICKPEAS

2 (14 oz) cans chickpeas
½ tbsp olive oil
1 tbsp smoked paprika
2 tsp ground cumin
2 tsp ground coriander
a pinch of salt

FOR THE SALAD

1 medium cucumber
9 oz cherry tomatoes
1 ripe avocado
1 lemon
16 fresh mint sprigs
1 tbsp extra-virgin olive oil
4 cups baby salad greens
salt and black pepper

FOR THE DRESSING

1 tbsp tahini
1 tbsp maple syrup
½ tbsp olive oil
½ tsp salt
2 tsp water

PREHEAT OVEN TO 350°F | LINE A SHEET PAN WITH PARCHMENT PAPER

First, make the spiced chickpeas | Drain and rinse the chickpeas, then pat them dry with paper towels | Tip the chickpeas into a mixing bowl along with the olive oil, smoked paprika, cumin, coriander, and salt and toss to combine | Tip the chickpeas onto the lined sheet pan, spread them out, put the pan in the oven, and roast the chickpeas for 25 minutes

Now, prep the rest of the salad | Trim and quarter the cucumber, then cut it into small chunks | Halve the cherry tomatoes | Halve and carefully pit the avocado by tapping the pit firmly with the heel of a knife so that it lodges in the pit, then twist and remove | Peel the avocado, then dice the flesh | Halve the lemon | Pick the mint leaves (discarding the stems) and roughly chop

Take the chickpeas out of the oven and tip them into a mixing bowl | Add the cucumber, cherry tomatoes, half the chopped mint leaves, and the avocado | Squeeze the juice from both lemon halves over the contents of the bowl, add the olive oil, and gently toss with salad servers to combine | Taste, season to perfection with salt and pepper, and gently toss again

Make the dressing | Mix all the ingredients in a small bowl until smooth

Add the baby salad greens to the bowl of dressing and toss to combine | Serve the salad in bowls, sprinkle over the remaining mint leaves, drizzle over the dressing, and eat immediately

345 KCAL | LOW SUGAR | FULL OF FIBER | PROTEIN PACKED

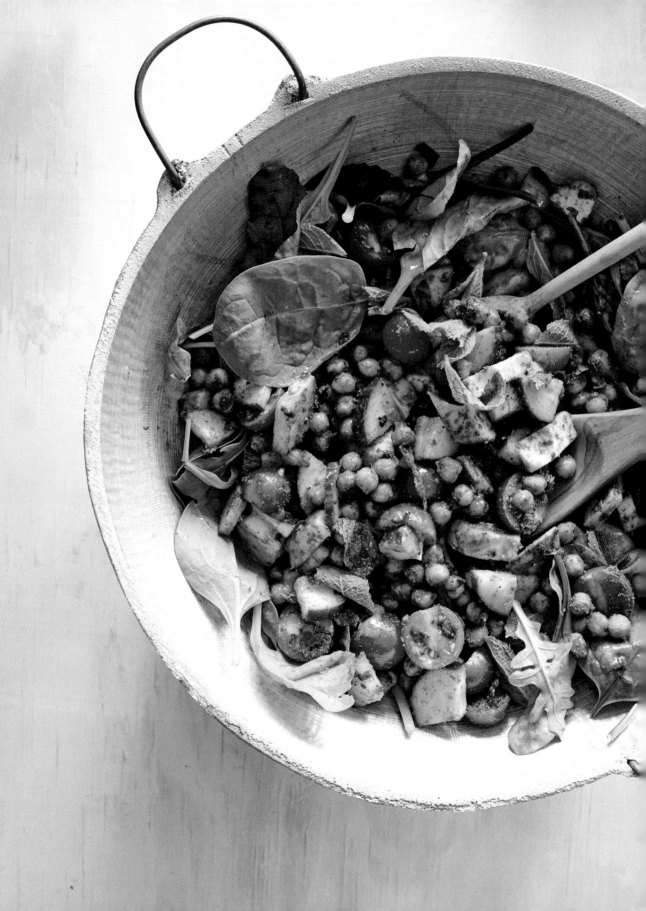

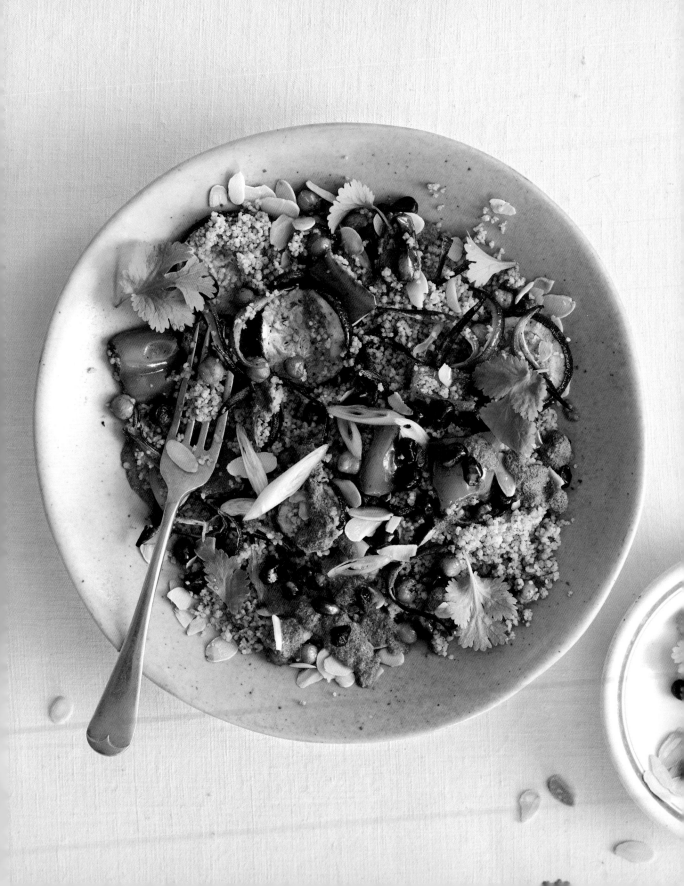

SALSA VERDE COUSCOUS

SERVES 2

FOR THE COUSCOUS

1 (14 oz) can chickpeas
½ tsp sumac
½ tsp maple syrup
1 red onion
1 zucchini
1 red bell pepper
2 tsp olive oil
¾ cup couscous
salt and black pepper

FOR THE SALSA VERDE

2 small fresh green chiles
2 garlic cloves
1½ cups fresh cilantro
2 cups fresh parsley
    leaves
⅓ cup fresh mint leaves
scant ½ cup fresh basil
    leaves
1 tbsp apple cider vinegar
1 tsp Dijon mustard
6–8 cornichons
½ tbsp capers
1 tbsp extra-virgin olive oil
3 tbsp water, plus
    extra if needed
1 lime
pinch of salt

TO GARNISH

2 tbsp sliced almonds
1 scallion
2 tbsp pomegranate
    seeds

Couscous is a great pantry ingredient for quick, easy meals. We've hit this one with citrusy, sumac-y flavors and tossed it with a salsa verde dressing and some roasted veg. It makes double the amount of salsa verde you need, so save the leftovers in a sealable container in the fridge for up to 5 days. Or double the couscous for your lunchbox the next day.

PREHEAT OVEN TO 375°F | LINE A SHEET PAN WITH PARCHMENT PAPER | BLENDER | BOILING WATER | SKILLET

First, prep and roast the chickpeas and vegetables | Drain and rinse the chickpeas and pat them dry with paper towels | Put the chickpeas in a bowl with the sumac and maple syrup and toss to coat

Peel and slice the red onion | Trim and slice the zucchini | Trim, halve, and core the bell pepper and cut it into small bite-sized chunks | Spread the vegetables and the chickpeas out on the lined sheet pan, drizzle with the olive oil, and season with salt and pepper | Put the pan in the oven and roast for 25 minutes

While the vegetables are roasting, make the salsa verde | Rip the stems from the chiles, cut them in half lengthwise, and remove the seeds if you prefer a milder salsa | Peel the garlic | Halve the limes and squeeze the lime juice into the blender | Put all the remaining salsa verde ingredients, apart from ¼ cup of cilantro leaves, in the blender and blitz to make a sauce | Taste and season to perfection with salt and pepper, and add a splash of water to loosen if necessary

Now, prep the couscous and the garnish | Cook the couscous in boiling water following the package instructions | Toast the almonds in a hot, dry skillet for a couple of minutes and set to one side | Trim and thinly slice the scallion

Serve the couscous | Add 2 tablespoons of the salsa verde to the couscous and fold to combine | Add the roasted vegetables to the bowl and fold them into the couscous | Plate up the Salsa Verde Couscous, garnish with the toasted almonds, scallion, reserved cilantro leaves, and pomegranate seeds | Drizzle over a little more salsa verde and serve

679 KCAL | LOW SUGAR | FULL OF FIBER | PROTEIN PACKED

RAINBOW STIR-FRY

SERVES 2

1 red onion
2-inch piece fresh ginger
1 red bell pepper
1½ oz lacinato kale
1¾ oz broccolini
1¾ oz baby corn
1 carrot
⅓ cup frozen shelled
    edamame
5 oz whole wheat noodles
½ tbsp canola oil
1 tsp sesame oil
2 oz snow peas
3 tbsp cashews, toasted
salt and black pepper

FOR THE SAUCE

3 garlic cloves
3 limes
1–2 fresh red Thai chiles
½ tbsp soy sauce
1 tsp sesame oil
1½ tbsp rice vinegar
1 cup fresh cilantro leaves

TO SERVE

4 radishes
1 scallion
1 lime
½ cup fresh cilantro
    leaves
1 tbsp mixed sesame
    seeds

This dish is exactly what we mean when we say to "eat the rainbow." Just look at all that color! It's a super-quick dish to cook, so get everything ready before you start. This stir-fry contains a few different sources of plant-based proteins, including edamame, noodles, and cashews, but to boost the protein even further, add a little tofu.

BLENDER | FINE GRATER OR MICROPLANE | SAUCEPAN | WOK

First, make the sauce | Peel and roughly chop the garlic | Halve the limes | Rip the stems from the chiles, cut them in half lengthwise, and remove the seeds if you wish | Put the garlic cloves, soy sauce, sesame oil, rice vinegar, chiles, and cilantro leaves into the blender | Squeeze the lime juice into the blender and blitz to make a sauce | Taste, tweak, and season to perfection with salt and pepper | Keep to one side

Now, prep the components of the stir-fry | Peel and thinly slice the red onion | Peel the ginger by scraping off the skin with a spoon, then grate | Trim, halve, and core the red bell pepper, then thinly slice | Remove the tough midribs from the kale and thinly slice the leaves | Trim and quarter the broccolini lengthwise | Halve the baby corn lengthwise | Peel the carrot and cut it into matchsticks | Cook the edamame following the package instructions

Trim and thinly slice the radishes | Trim and thinly slice the scallion | Cut the lime into wedges

Now, prep the noodles | Cook the noodles following the package instructions | Drain the noodles in a colander, tip them back into the saucepan, pour over the sauce, and toss to combine

Time to make your stir-fry | Heat the canola oil in the wok over high heat | Add the red onion, ginger, bell pepper, and a pinch of salt and stir (or toss) for 1 minute | Add the broccolini and baby corn and stir for 1 minute | Add the kale, edamame, and sesame oil and stir for 1 minute | Add the carrot and snow peas and stir for 1 minute | Tip the cooked noodles into the pan and stir for 1 minute

Time to serve | Plate up the stir-fry, sprinkle it with the cashews, radishes, scallion, cilantro leaves, and sesame seeds, and serve immediately with the lime wedges

539 KCAL | LOW SUGAR | FULL OF FIBER | PROTEIN PACKED

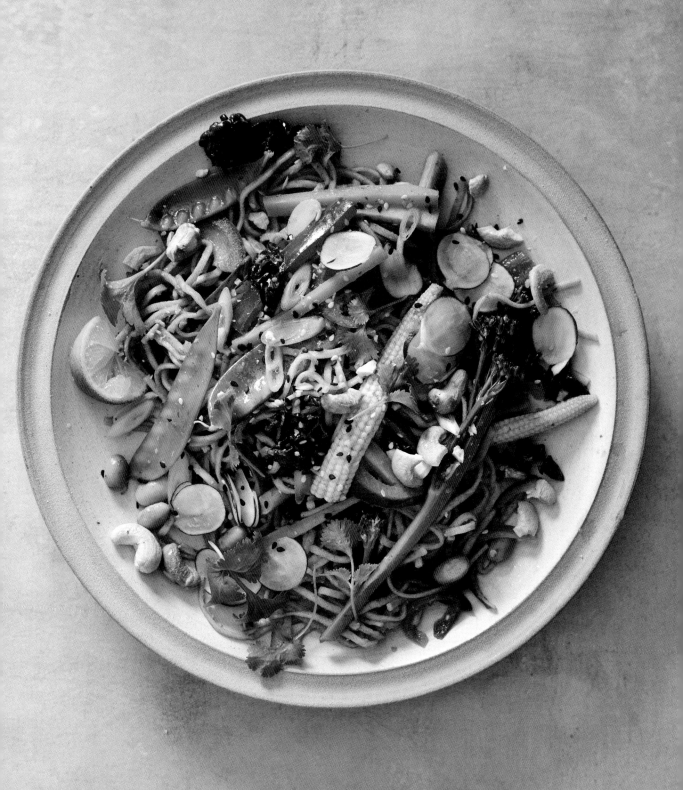

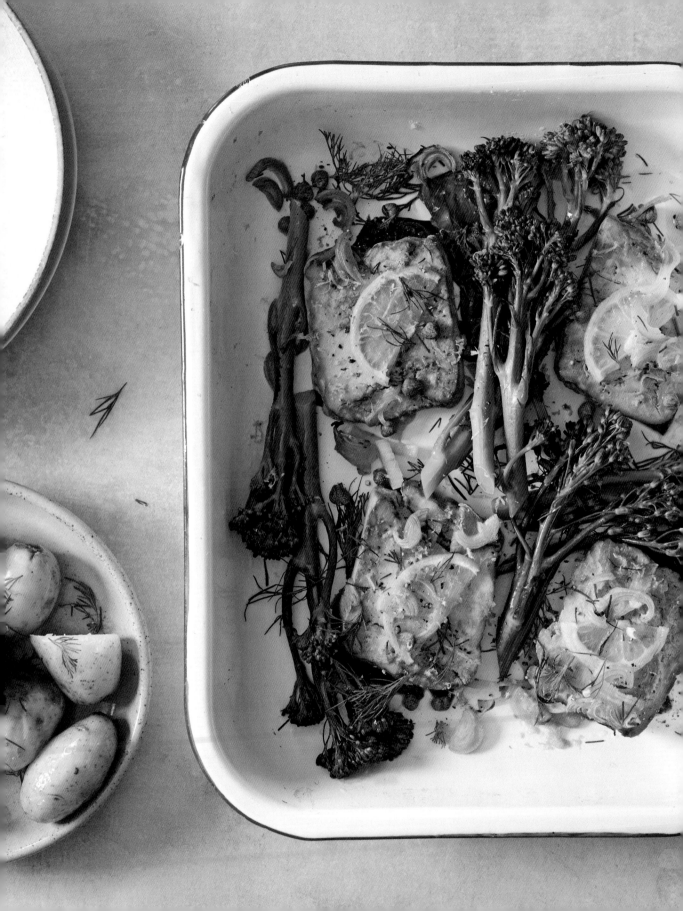

OVEN-ROASTED "SALMON" TOFU STEAKS

Tofu is such a great and versatile ingredient and is now the main component of many of our favorite dishes. In our pre-vegan days, a common post-gym health food for us was salmon and steamed veg, so we set about re-creating salmon using tofu. With the addition of beets, we think we've cracked it!

SERVES 2

9 oz firm tofu

3 tbsp beet juice

2 nori sheets

1 shallot

1 tbsp capers, plus 1 tbsp caper brine

2 lemons

1 cup fresh dill sprigs, plus a sprinkling to serve, optional

1 tbsp olive oil

3 tbsp white wine

10 oz new potatoes

7 oz broccolini

salt and black pepper

PREHEAT OVEN TO 350°F | TOFU PRESS OR 2 CLEAN TEA TOWELS AND A WEIGHT SUCH AS A HEAVY BOOK | SCISSORS | LINE A SHEET PAN WITH PARCHMENT PAPER | PASTRY BRUSH | SAUCEPAN

Press the tofu using a tofu press or place it between two clean tea towels, lay it on a plate, and put a weight on top | Leave for at least 30 minutes to drain off any liquid and firm up

Cut the block of tofu lengthwise into 4 equal-sized slices, pour the beet juice into the bowl, put the slices of tofu in the bowl, and leave to marinate for 3–4 minutes while you prep the other ingredients

Cut the nori with scissors into 4 squares that match the shape of the 4 slices of tofu | Peel and finely chop the shallot | Finely chop the capers | Zest and juice one of the lemons, cut 2 slices out of the second lemon, and cut the slices in half | Pick and roughly chop the dill leaves | Take the tofu out of the bowl of beet juice and pat it dry with paper towels

Lay the nori on the sheet pan | Lay one piece of tofu on each piece of nori | Add the lemon zest and juice, dill, capers, caper brine, shallot, and white wine | Cover the pan completely with foil, put the pan in the oven, and bake for 20 minutes

While the tofu is baking, cook the potatoes | Halve any larger potatoes, so they are roughly the same size as the smaller ones | Place the new potatoes in a saucepan of lightly salted water, bring to a boil, and simmer for 15 minutes, or until tender | Drain the potatoes and season to taste with salt and pepper and garnish with dill, if you like

Take the tofu out of the oven, remove the foil, lay the broccolini in the gaps between the tofu, and put the pan back in the oven for another 10 minutes

Remove the pan from the oven, plate up the tofu "salmon," broccolini, and potatoes and serve immediately

427 KCAL | LOW SUGAR | FULL OF FIBER | PROTEIN PACKED

GREEN SHAKSHUKA

This gorgeously green pot of goodness uses plant-based yogurt in place of traditional eggs. Za'atar is a blend of dried herbs, and it is a wonderful way to add a Middle Eastern flavor to any dish, while the combo of fresh mint, dill, and parsley keeps it tasting light and clean. Packed with sources of vitamins A, B5, B6, C, E, and K, folate, potassium, manganese, and thiamine, while being high in protein and fiber—trust us, this one is good for you!

SERVES 2

1 leek
2 garlic cloves
1 (14 oz) can cannellini beans
½ cup fresh mint leaves
½ cup fresh parsley leaves
½ cup fresh dill
1 ripe avocado
1 tbsp olive oil
1½ cups frozen peas
7 oz fresh spinach leaves
3½ tbsp plant-based yogurt
½ tsp za'atar
salt and black pepper
4 slices crusty whole wheat bread, to serve

FINE GRATER OR MICROPLANE | LARGE SKILLET

First, prep your ingredients | Trim and thinly slice the leek | Peel and grate the garlic | Drain and rinse the cannellini beans | Roughly chop the mint, parsley, and dill | Halve and carefully pit the avocado by tapping the pit firmly with the heel of a knife so that it lodges in the pit, then twist and remove | Scoop out and slice the avocado flesh

Now, start cooking | Heat the olive oil in the large skillet over medium-high heat | Add the leek and cook, stirring, for 5 minutes, until softened | Turn down the heat, add the garlic, and stir for another minute | Add the beans and peas and stir for 2 minutes | Add the spinach, one handful at a time, stirring constantly and allowing each batch of spinach to wilt down before adding the next

Time to plate up | When all the spinach has wilted and the peas are thoroughly thawed and cooked through, take the pan off the heat, stir in the mint, parsley, and dill, and season to perfection with salt and pepper | Top with the yogurt, za'atar, and the sliced avocado, and serve with crusty whole wheat bread

616 KCAL | LOW SUGAR | FULL OF FIBER | PROTEIN PACKED

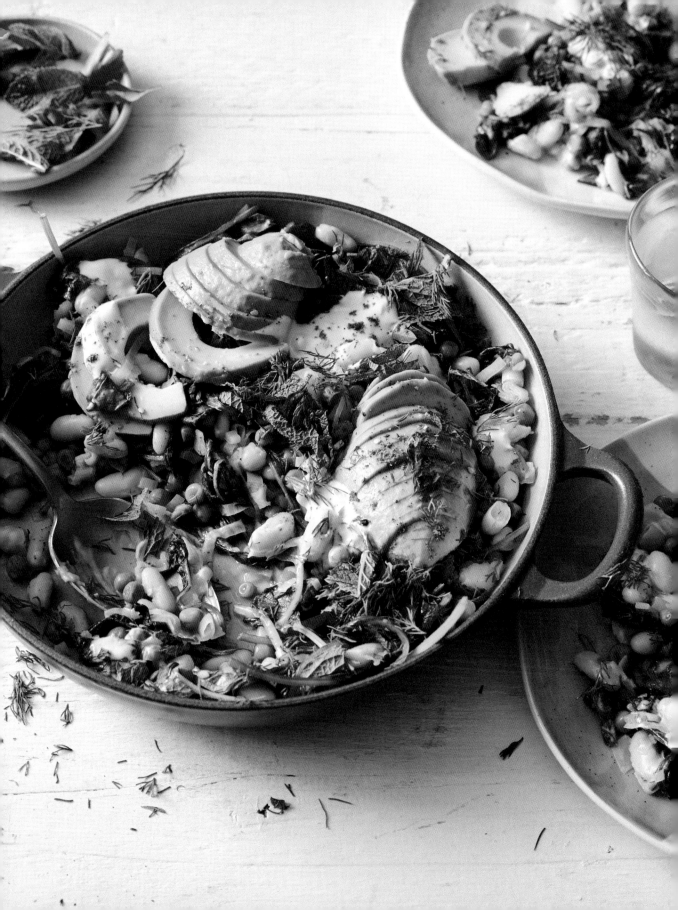

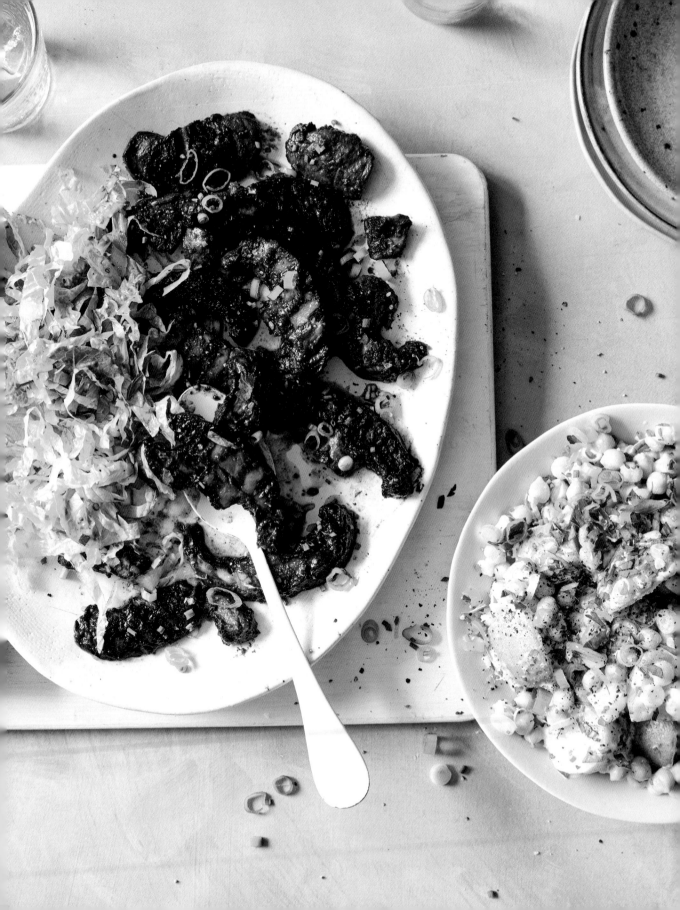

BBQ PORTOBELLO & POTATO SALAD

This is a fantastic, light summer evening dinner. The BBQ mushrooms are succulent, smoky, and incredibly satisfying, and they work perfectly with the protein-packed chickpea potato salad. Our lower-sugar BBQ sauce also makes a delicious condiment, so batch the sauce to use in other dishes.

SERVES 2

SAUCEPAN | FINE GRATER OR MICROPLANE | GRILL PAN

FOR THE POTATO & CHICKPEA SALAD

10 oz new potatoes

½ oz fresh chives

¾ cup fresh parsley leaves

4 scallions

1 (14 oz) can chickpeas

3 tbsp vegan mayonnaise

1 tbsp white wine vinegar

2 lemons

salt and black pepper

FOR THE BBQ MUSHROOMS

1 tbsp olive oil

4 tbsp BBQ sauce (low-sugar store-bought or use our BBQ Bourbon Sauce on page 169)

1 tbsp smoked paprika

1 tsp garlic powder

½ tsp cayenne pepper

1 tsp onion powder

4 portobello mushrooms

salt and black pepper

½ head romaine lettuce (about 5 oz), to serve

First, make the potato salad | Put the new potatoes in the saucepan (make sure they're roughly the same size, cutting bigger ones in half if necessary), cover with cold water, add a pinch of salt, put the pan over high heat, and bring to a boil | Simmer for 8–10 minutes, until the potatoes are tender

While the potatoes are cooking, finely chop the chives and parsley, trim and finely chop the scallions, and put them in a bowl | Drain and rinse the chickpeas and add to the bowl | Add the mayonnaise and white wine vinegar and stir to combine | Halve the lemons | Zest one of the lemons and squeeze the juice | Add to the bowl of mayonnaise, stir, and season to perfection with salt and pepper

Drain the potatoes and run them under cold water in a colander to help them cool slightly | Leave to drain, then add them to the bowl and fold until the potatoes are well coated in the mayonnaise mixture | Set the bowl to one side

Now, make the BBQ mushrooms | Put the olive oil, BBQ sauce, smoked paprika, garlic powder, cayenne pepper, onion powder, and a pinch each of salt and pepper in a bowl and mix with a fork to make a marinade | Reserve ½ tablespoon of the marinade in a separate cup | Add a splash of boiling water to the bowl and stir to combine

Cut the mushrooms into slices 1 inch thick, add them to the bowl, and stir to combine, making sure they're well coated in the mixture | Put the grill pan over medium heat, and when it is hot, add the mushrooms and cook for 3–4 minutes on each side | Remove the mushrooms from the heat and toss them gently with the remaining sauce

Plate up | Shred the lettuce and divide it between plates, squeezing over some of the juice from the remaining two lemon halves | Divide the potato salad and BBQ mushrooms between the plates and serve immediately

531 KCAL | LOW FAT | LOW SUGAR | FULL OF FIBER | PROTEIN PACKED

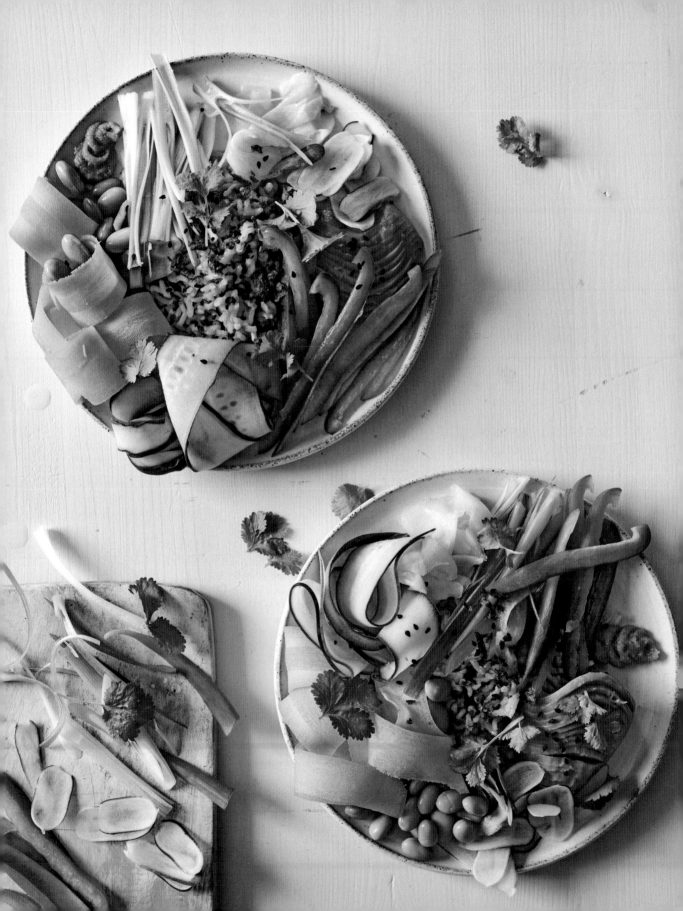

SUPER SUSHI SALAD

Sushi is a favorite grab-and-go meal of ours, and a variation of it has appeared in both our previous cookbooks. However, it can be a bit time-consuming to make, so we decided to deconstruct it here to save time. We've used a rainbow spread of colorful vegetables served with deliciously soured brown rice, wasabi, sesame seeds, and pickled ginger.

SERVES 4

⅔ cup frozen shelled edamame
1 medium cucumber
1 large carrot
4 scallions
6 radishes
1 red bell pepper
1 ripe avocado
½ cup fresh cilantro leaves
1½ tbsp pickled ginger
salt and black pepper

FOR THE RICE

1 nori sheet
2 (8.8 oz) bags microwaveable brown basmati rice
1 tbsp mirin
2 tbsp soy sauce
1 tbsp wasabi

TO SERVE

2 tbsp wasabi, optional
1 tsp black sesame seeds

SAUCEPAN | VEGETABLE PEELER | BLENDER

First, prepare the ingredients | Cook the edamame following the instructions on the package | Trim and peel the cucumber into long ribbons using a vegetable peeler | Peel the carrot, then use the vegetable peeler to peel it into long ribbons | Trim, halve, and thinly slice the scallions lengthwise | Trim and thinly slice the radishes | Trim, halve, core, and thinly slice the red bell pepper | Halve and carefully pit the avocado by tapping the pit firmly with the heel of a knife so that it lodges in the pit, then twist and remove | Scoop out the avocado flesh and thinly slice it | Blitz the nori sheet in the blender (or slice it into small shards with a sharp knife) | Cook the rice following the instructions on the package and leave to cool slightly

Now, season the rice | Put the mirin, soy sauce, and wasabi in a mixing bowl with half the nori | Add the rice and toss to combine | Taste the rice and season to perfection with salt and pepper

Time to plate up | Fluff the rice and divide it among plates | Creatively plate up all the prepared vegetables | Dress the servings with cilantro leaves, pickled ginger, the remaining nori, spots of wasabi (if using), and a sprinkle of sesame seeds and serve immediately

372 KCAL | LOW SUGAR | FULL OF FIBER | PROTEIN PACKED

JERK JACKFRUIT SALAD 'N' BEANS

SERVES 4

2 (14 oz) cans young green jackfruit in water

4 cups cooked basmati rice or 2 (8.8 oz) bags microwavable brown basmati rice

salt and black pepper

FOR THE JERK-STYLE SPICE PASTE

1 garlic clove

1¼-inch piece fresh ginger

2 scallions

1 Scotch bonnet chile

½ cup fresh parsley

½ cup fresh cilantro

1 tbsp ground allspice

1 tbsp ground black pepper

1 tbsp chile flakes

½ tbsp muscovado sugar

½ tbsp maple syrup

2 tbsp water

1 tbsp olive oil

FOR THE DRESSING

1 lime

1 garlic clove

1 fresh red chile

1 tbsp extra-virgin olive oil

FOR THE SALAD 'N' BEANS

1 red bell pepper

1 large tomato

½ red onion

3½ oz fresh mango

1 (14 oz) can mixed beans

2½ tbsp cashews

¾ cup fresh cilantro leaves

In 2017 we created a jerk jackfruit video with AllPlants, which makes tasty plant-based ready-meals. Jackfruit is now much more readily available. Our own jerk seasoning adds fire and complex spice, and the mango, beans, and cashew provide extra flavor and nutrition to this surprisingly easy dinner.

PREHEAT OVEN TO 350°F | LINE A SHEET PAN WITH PARCHMENT PAPER | SMALL FOOD PROCESSOR | FINE GRATER OR MICROPLANE

First, make the spice paste | Peel the garlic | Peel the ginger by scraping off the skin with a spoon | Trim and roughly chop the scallions | Rip the stem from the Scotch bonnet chile, cut in half lengthwise, remove the seeds, and roughly chop | Put the garlic, ginger, scallions, Scotch bonnet, parsley, cilantro (leaves and stems), allspice, black pepper, chile flakes, muscovado sugar, maple syrup, water, and olive oil in the food processor and blitz to form a coarse paste

Now, prep the jackfruit | Drain the jackfruit, rinse under a cold tap, and pat dry with a clean tea towel or paper towels | Lay the jackfruit out on a cutting board and pull it into pieces with two forks | Pat dry with paper towels once more | Transfer the pulled jackfruit to a mixing bowl, add the spice paste, and mix well | Tip the spiced jackfruit out onto the lined sheet pan, making sure the pieces are evenly spaced apart | Put the pan in the oven and roast the jackfruit for 30 minutes

Now, prep the dressing | Halve the lime | Peel and grate the garlic | Rip the stem from the chile, cut it in half lengthwise, remove the seeds, and finely dice | Squeeze the juice from the lime into a mug | Add the garlic, chile, olive oil, and a pinch each of salt and pepper to the mug and stir well to combine

Prep the salad 'n' beans | Trim, halve, core, and dice the bell pepper | Dice the tomato | Peel and finely dice the red onion | Dice the mango flesh | Drain and rinse the beans | Roughly chop the cashews

Put the beans, pepper, tomato, red onion, mango, cashews, cilantro leaves, and dressing in a bowl and toss to combine | Taste the salad and season to perfection with salt and pepper

Time to assemble the dish | Heat the rice, if necessary, or cook it following the package instructions, and transfer to serving bowls | Spread the jackfruit over the rice | Dress the bowls with the salad and serve immediately

543 KCAL | LOW FAT | LOW SUGAR | FULL OF FIBER

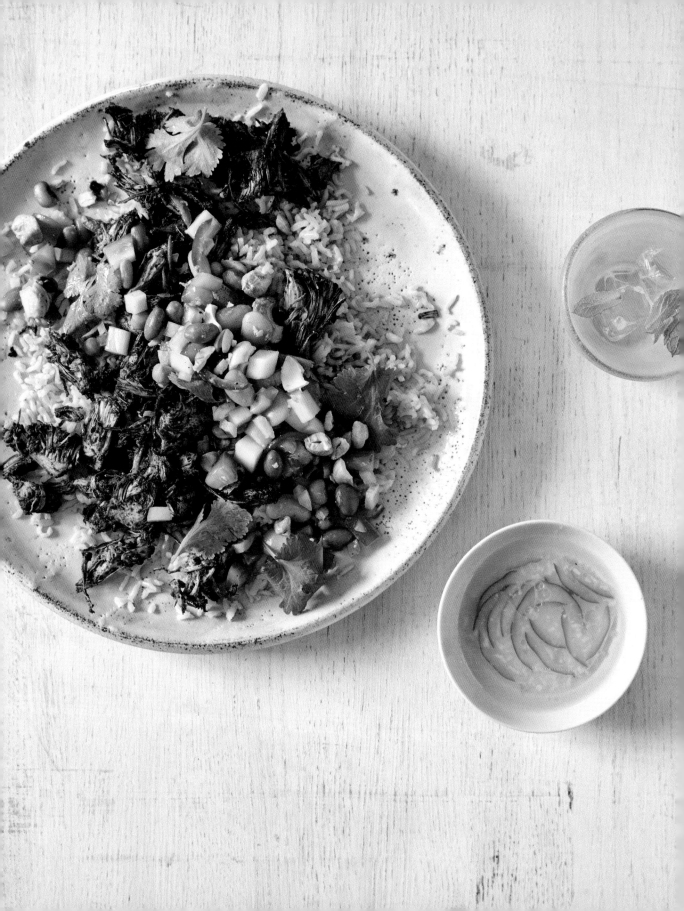

THAI TEMPEH SALAD

We predict tempeh will be the next hot new ingredient. It's a good source of protein, made from fermented soybeans, while being healthier and less processed than tofu. It's thought to be great for the gut, and is a good source of fiber and iron and a bunch of other nutrients. Tempeh takes on flavor really well, and is easy to cook. An all-round winner! Here we've used a delicious mix of Thai flavors in a quick, easy-to-assemble salad.

SERVES 2

PREHEAT OVEN TO 350°F | SAUCEPAN | STEAMER | FINE GRATER OR MICROPLANE | OVENPROOF DISH | VEGETABLE PEELER

FOR THE MARINATED TEMPEH

7 oz tempeh

2 garlic cloves

2¾-inch piece fresh ginger

4 limes

1 or 2 Thai red chiles

1 tbsp soy sauce

3 tbsp apple juice

2 tbsp rice vinegar

1 tbsp sesame oil

FOR THE SALAD

1 carrot

½ cucumber

2 scallions

¼ red cabbage

2 oz snow peas

10 cherry tomatoes

3 tbsp unsalted peanuts

1½ cups fresh cilantro leaves

salt and black pepper

First, prep the tempeh | Cut the tempeh into bite-sized pieces | Half-fill the saucepan with water and bring to a boil | Add the tempeh to the steamer, place over the pan of boiling water, put the lid on, and steam the tempeh for 8–10 minutes

Now, make the marinade | Peel and grate the garlic | Peel the ginger by scraping off the skin with a spoon, then grate it | Zest and juice the limes | Trim and finely dice the red chile(s) | Put the garlic, ginger, lime zest and juice, chile, soy sauce, apple juice, rice vinegar, and sesame oil in a mixing bowl and stir to combine | Transfer half the marinade to a small bowl and set to one side until ready to serve

Cook the tempeh | Place the tempeh pieces in the ovenproof dish, pour over the marinade in the mixing bowl, stir the tempeh to coat, put the dish in the oven, and bake for 20 minutes

While the tempeh is in the oven, prep the salad | Peel the carrot, then peel it lengthwise into long ribbons using the vegetable peeler | Trim the cucumber and peel it lengthwise into long ribbons | Trim and thinly slice the scallions | Thinly slice the red cabbage and snow peas | Halve the cherry tomatoes | Roughly chop the peanuts | Roughly chop the fresh cilantro

Build the salad | Combine all the salad ingredients and the baked tempeh in a bowl and toss with the remaining marinade and the cilantro | Season to taste with salt and pepper and serve immediately

371 KCAL | LOW FAT | LOW SUGAR | FULL OF FIBER | PROTEIN PACKED

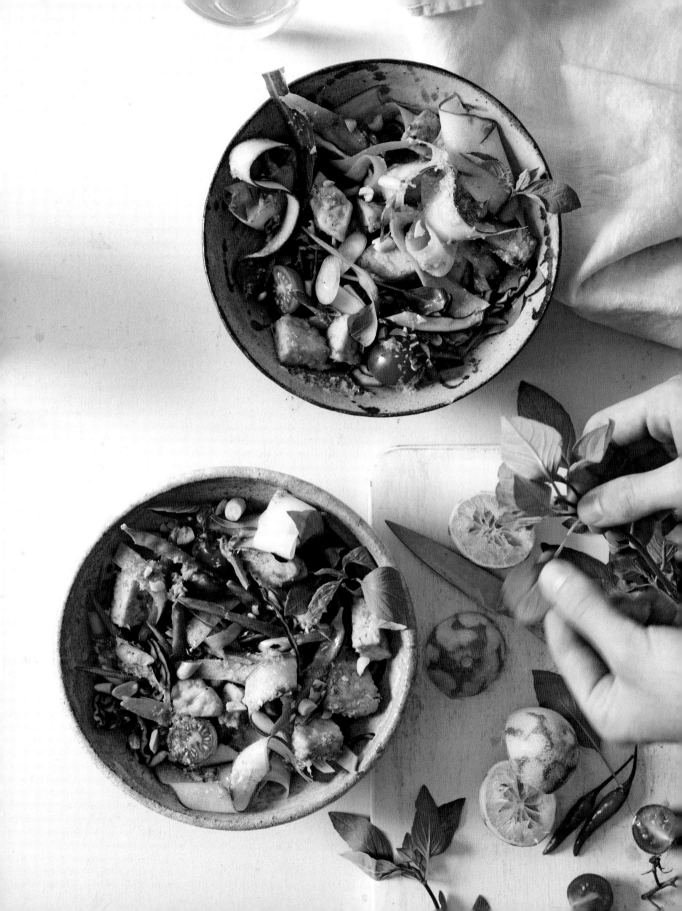

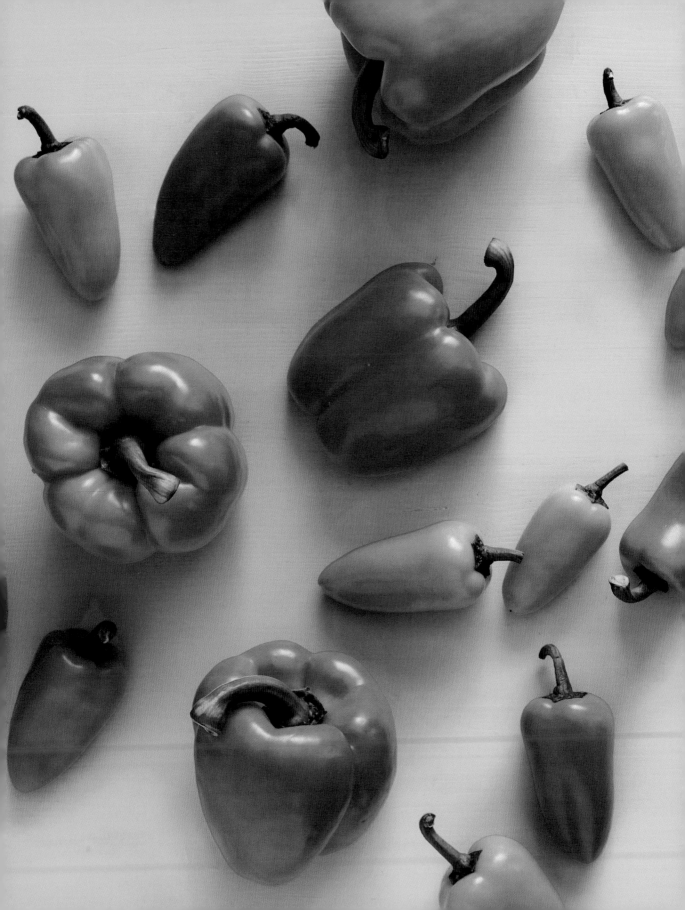

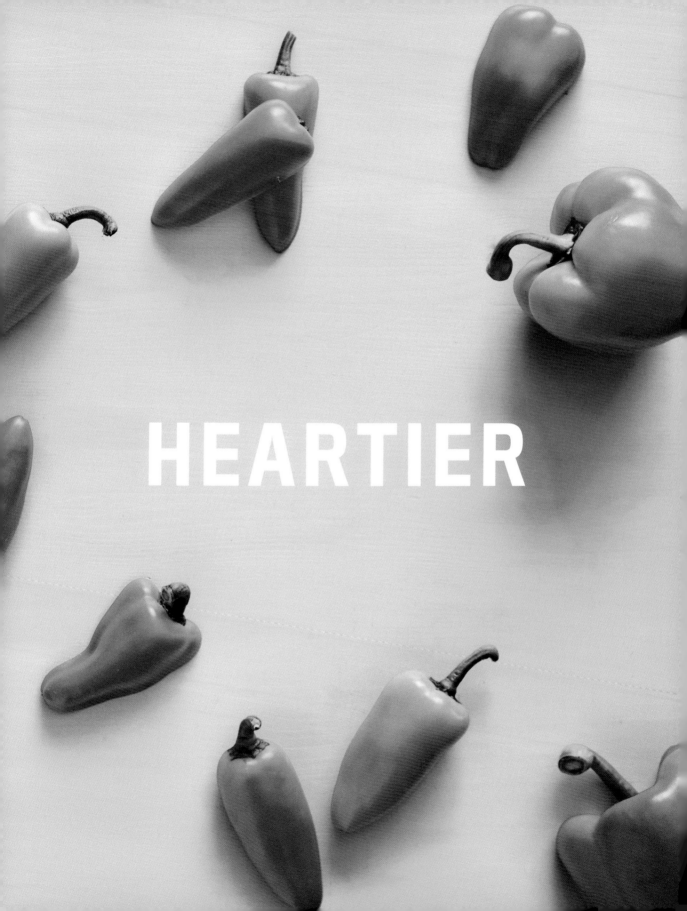

HEARTIER

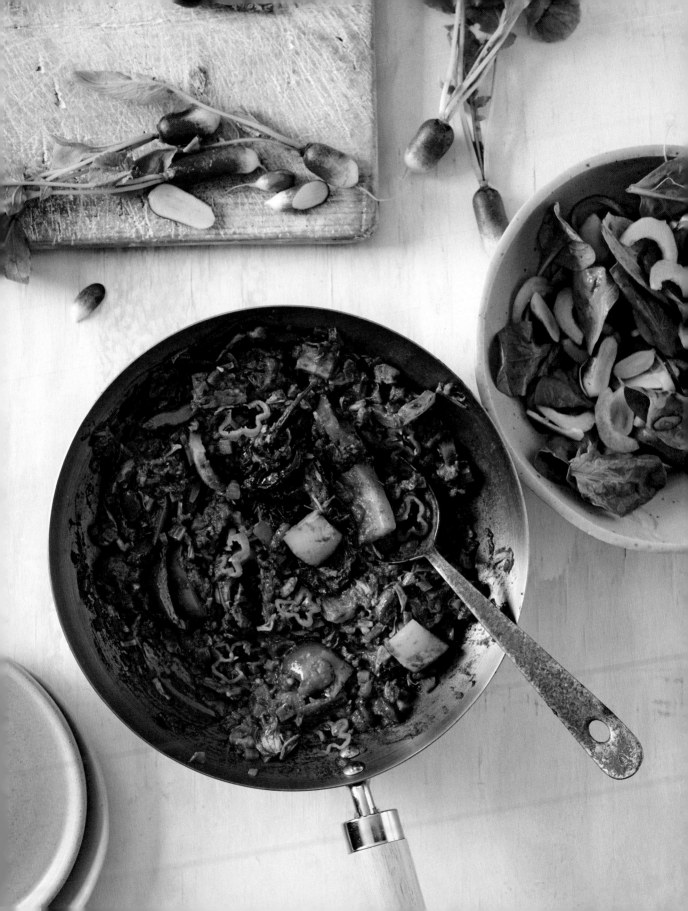

BRAISED JACK CHILI

SERVES 4

FOR THE SPICE MIX

2 tsp chili powder
½ tsp salt
2 tsp ground cumin
1 tsp dried oregano
¼ tsp ground allspice
¼ tsp ground cinnamon

FOR THE CHILI

1 (14 oz) can young green
   jackfruit in water
2 red onions
1 celery stalk
1 carrot
6 garlic cloves
1 red bell pepper
1 yellow bell pepper
2 fresh red chiles
1 (14 oz) can kidney beans
⅓ cup walnuts
1 tbsp olive oil, plus
   extra for drizzling
pinch of salt
1 (28 oz) can whole peeled
   tomatoes
1 bay leaf
1 dried ancho chile
   (about 6g), optional
1 oz dark chocolate
2 tsp soy sauce
½ cup water

TO SERVE

4 cups cooked basmati
   rice or 2 (8.8 oz) bags
   microwaveable brown
   basmati rice
1 lime
3½ oz mixed salad greens

One of our favorite street food spots in London is Biff's Jack Shack—and we kindly asked his permission to create our own version of his incredible braised jackfruit chili. Our quick version cheats a little bit—we simply flavor then roast the jackfruit. Then we make a delicious rich chili!

PREHEAT OVEN TO 425°F | LINE A SHEET PAN | FINE GRATER OR MICROPLANE | LARGE SAUCEPAN OR WOK

First, prep the jackfruit | Mix all the spice mix ingredients together in a small bowl | Drain the jackfruit, rinse under a cold tap, and pat dry with a clean tea towel or paper towels | Put the jackfruit on a cutting board and use two forks to pull it apart into pieces | Pat the jackfruit dry again | Transfer the jackfruit pieces to the lined sheet pan | Drizzle with a little olive oil, sprinkle over half of the spice mix, and mix to coat | Put the pan in the oven and roast the jackfruit for 20–30 minutes

Now, make the chili | Peel and finely chop the red onions | Trim and thinly slice the celery | Peel and dice the carrot (use a food processor to chop the vegetables if you like) | Peel and grate the garlic | Trim, halve, and core the bell peppers and cut them into bite-sized chunks | Rip the stems from the chiles and thinly slice (remove the seeds if you prefer) | Drain and rinse the kidney beans | Roughly chop the walnuts

Heat the olive oil in the large saucepan or wok over medium heat | Add the onions and the pinch of salt and stir for 3–4 minutes | Add the garlic and stir for 1 minute | Add the celery and carrot and cook, stirring, for 3 minutes | Add the remaining spice mix and stir for 30 seconds | Add the bell peppers and chiles and stir for 3–4 minutes | Add the walnuts, roasted jackfruit, tomatoes, bay leaf, ancho chile (if using), dark chocolate, drained kidney beans, soy sauce, and the water to the pan or wok | Reduce the heat and leave the chili to simmer and thicken for 12–15 minutes

Time to serve | Remove the ancho chile and bay leaf from the pan or wok | Prepare the rice | Cut the lime into wedges | Serve the chili over the rice, with a small side salad and lime wedges

582 KCAL | LOW FAT | LOW SUGAR | FULL OF FIBER | PROTEIN PACKED

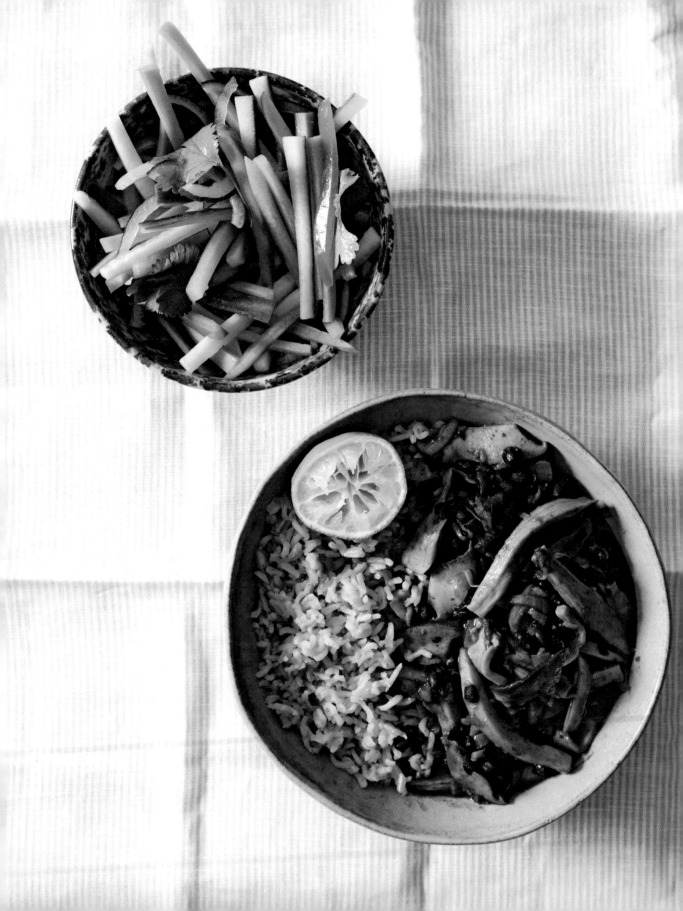

FEIJOADA & SLAW

SERVES 2

2 cups cooked basmati rice or 1 (8.8 oz) bag microwavable brown basmati rice

1 lime

salt and black pepper

FOR THE BASE

7 oz king oyster mushrooms (3 large)

1 large red onion

2 garlic cloves

½ fresh red chile

2 sprigs fresh rosemary

1 tbsp olive oil

1 tsp yeast extract (e.g., Marmite)

1 tsp soy sauce

FOR THE STEW

1 (14 oz) can black beans

¾ cup water

1 tbsp maple syrup

½ tsp cayenne pepper

1 tsp smoked paprika

2 bay leaves

¼ tsp ground cinnamon

1 tsp ground coriander

7 tbsp oat cream

FOR THE SLAW

1 small carrot (about 2½ oz)

1 small cucumber (about 6 oz)

1 red bell pepper

½ small red onion

½ tsp sesame oil

1 tsp soy sauce

1 tsp rice vinegar

½ tsp maple syrup

½ lime

¼ cup fresh cilantro leaves, plus extra to serve

Liam Chau, from High Grade Coffee in London, came to cook with us and showed us his favorite dish, feijoada. The flavors are deep, rich, and smoky, and the king oyster mushrooms give it an incredible meatiness, but you can use shiitake, oyster, or portobello instead if you like.

FINE GRATER OR MICROPLANE | SOUP POT

First, prep the ingredients for the base | Cut the caps off the mushrooms and thinly slice them | Shred the mushroom stalks into strands with two forks | Peel and finely chop the red onion | Peel and grate the garlic | Remove the seeds from the half chile and thinly slice | Pick the rosemary leaves from the sprigs and finely chop

Now, cook the base | Heat the olive oil in the soup pot over medium-low heat | Add the onion and a pinch of salt and cook, stirring, for 4–5 minutes | Add the garlic and chile and stir for 3–4 minutes | Add the yeast extract and stir again, then add the king oyster mushrooms and diced rosemary and stir for 5–10 minutes | Add the soy sauce and stir for 2 minutes

Now, finish the stew | Add the can of black beans to the pot, including the aquafaba (bean water), then half-fill the can with the ¾ cup water and set to one side | Add the maple syrup, cayenne pepper, smoked paprika, bay leaves, cinnamon, and coriander to the pot and stir for 2 minutes | Add the oat cream and the water from the can to the pot | Season to perfection with salt and pepper | Increase the temperature slightly and cook for 10–12 minutes, stirring very regularly to prevent the stew catching on the bottom of the pan

Now, for the slaw | Peel the carrot and cut it into matchsticks | Trim and halve the cucumber lengthwise, scoop out the watery seeds, and cut it into matchsticks | Trim, halve, core, and thinly slice the red bell pepper | Peel and thinly slice the red onion

Put the sesame oil, soy sauce, rice vinegar, and maple syrup in a mixing bowl, squeeze the juice from the half lime into the bowl and stir to combine | Add the carrot, cucumber, red pepper, and red onion to the bowl and toss to coat in the dressing | Sprinkle over the cilantro leaves and set to one side | Heat the rice, if necessary, or cook it following the package instructions

Time to serve | Halve the remaining lime | Plate up the rice, top with the feijoada and slaw, garnish with more cilantro leaves, and serve immediately, with the lime halves for squeezing

614 KCAL | LOW FAT | LOW SUGAR | FULL OF FIBER | PROTEIN PACKED

HEARTY, HERBY STEW

This warming dish makes for a perfect winter meal, and there's no need for any extra rice or breads as it's so filling. It is high in protein from the beans and lentils, and the huge amounts of fresh herbs add an extra healthy boost of flavor and nutrients. A serving of this will give you a good dose of vitamin C, K, A, folate, and iron in your diet.

SERVES 2

3 echalions (banana shallots) (about 3½ oz)

2 large garlic cloves

2 carrots

1 celery stalk

8 sprigs fresh thyme

2 sprigs fresh rosemary

4 fresh sage leaves

9 oz new potatoes

1 (14 oz) can green lentils

1 (14 oz) can cannellini beans

7 oz lacinato kale

¾ cup fresh parsley leaves

1 lemon

1½ tbsp olive oil

3 tbsp white wine

1 cup vegetable stock

2 cups water

1 bay leaf

2 tsp Dijon mustard

1 tsp yeast extract (e.g., Marmite)

2 tbsp nutritional yeast

salt and black pepper

FINE GRATER OR MICROPLANE | SOUP POT

Prep the ingredients | Peel and finely dice the shallots | Peel and grate the garlic | Peel and finely chop the carrots | Trim and thinly slice the celery | Pick the thyme and rosemary leaves from the sprigs and finely chop | Thinly slice the sage leaves | Slice any larger potatoes so they are all a similar size | Drain and rinse the green lentils and cannellini beans | Remove the tough midribs from the kale and shred the leaves | Roughly chop the parsley | Halve the lemon

Heat the olive oil in the soup pot over medium heat | Add the shallots, carrots, and celery and a pinch of salt to the pan and cook, stirring, for 4–5 minutes | Add the garlic and stir for 1 minute | Add the thyme and rosemary and stir for another minute | Add the wine and simmer for 1 minute | Add the vegetable stock, water, bay leaf, and mustard and bring to a gentle simmer | Add the new potatoes | Cook for 12–15 minutes, until the potatoes are tender, then taste and season to perfection with salt and pepper

Add the lentils and cannellini beans to the stew, along with the juice of half the lemon, and simmer for 3–4 minutes | Add the kale, sage, yeast extract, and two-thirds of the parsley and stir for 2 minutes | Taste the stew, check the tenderness of the potatoes, and season again with salt and pepper

Serve up the stew | Ladle the stew into bowls and squeeze over lemon juice to taste | Sprinkle with the nutritional yeast and the remaining parsley and serve immediately

590 KCAL | LOW FAT | LOW SUGAR | FULL OF FIBER | PROTEIN PACKED

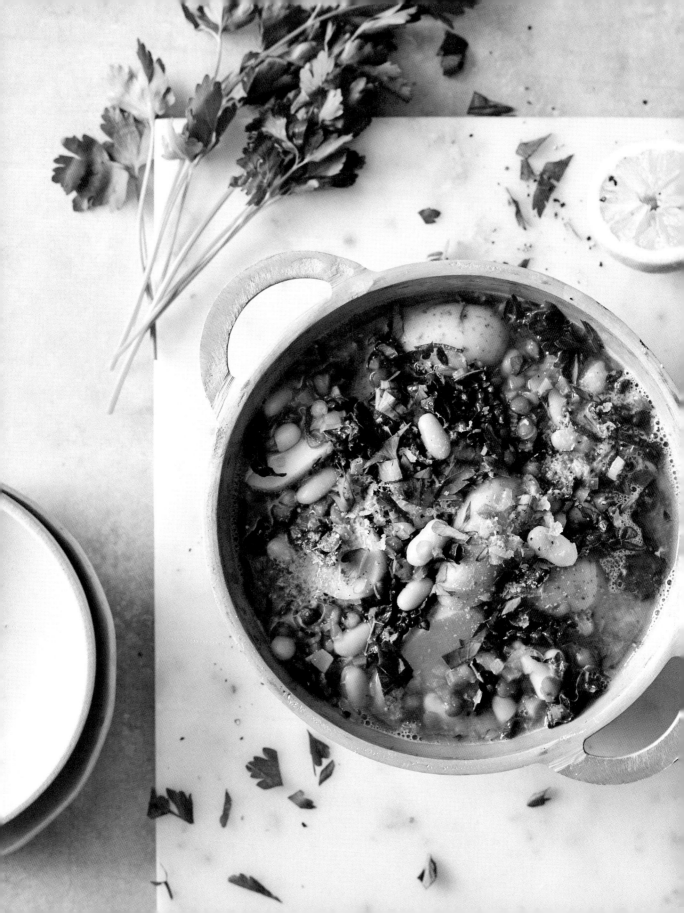

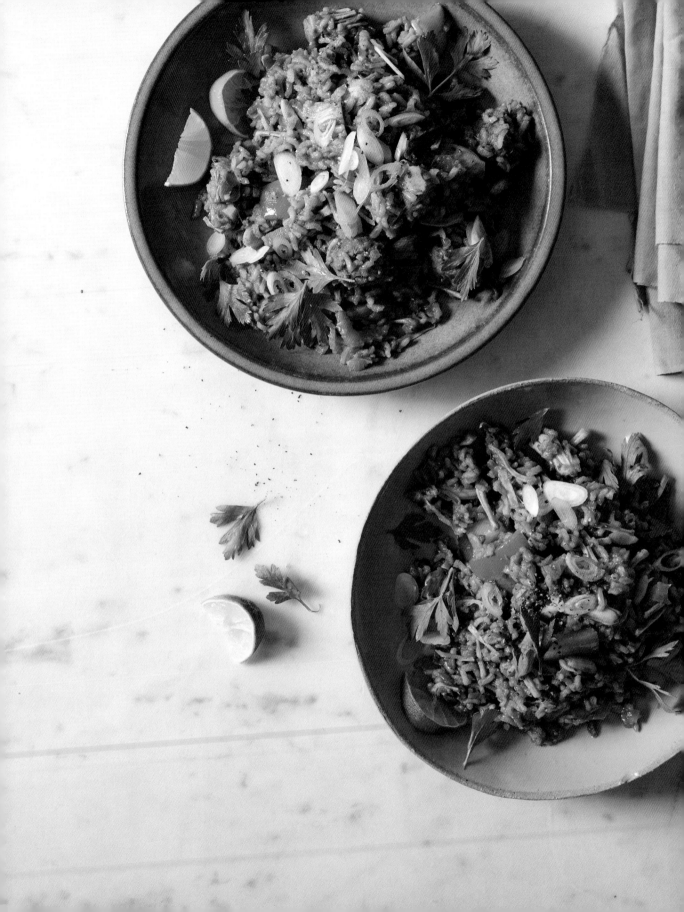

JAMMIN' JAMBALAYA

A jambalaya is a popular Creole dish that has roots in Mediterranean and African cuisines. Combining spices like this helps create a complex flavor throughout the whole dish. Using lots of different spices also means you'll benefit from the wide range of antioxidants that each spice contains.

SERVES 4

2 vegan sausages

1 (14 oz) can young green jackfruit in water or brine

4 sun-dried tomatoes, plus 1 tbsp oil from the jar

1 onion

1 red bell pepper

1 yellow bell pepper

1 celery stalk

3 garlic cloves

10 sprigs fresh thyme

2 (8.8 oz) bags microwaveable brown basmati rice

1 lime

2 tsp smoked paprika

½ tsp cayenne pepper

½ tsp dried oregano

1 tbsp tomato paste

1 (14 oz) can cherry tomatoes

¾ cup water

1 bay leaf

½ tsp hot sauce (e.g., Tabasco), plus extra to taste

4 scallions

¼ cup fresh parsley leaves

salt and black pepper

PREHEAT OVEN TO 350°F | LINE A SHEET PAN WITH PARCHMENT PAPER | FINE GRATER OR MICROPLANE | LARGE SAUCEPAN

First, prep the ingredients | Place the vegan sausages on the lined sheet pan, put the pan in the oven, and cook for 20 minutes | Drain the jackfruit, rinse under a cold tap, and pat dry with a clean tea towel or paper towels, then roughly chop | Thinly slice the sun-dried tomatoes | Peel and finely dice the onion | Trim, halve, and core the bell peppers and cut them into 1-inch chunks | Trim and thinly slice the celery | Peel and grate the garlic | Remove the thyme leaves from the sprigs | Cook the rice following the package instructions | Cut the lime in half

Fire up the stove and start cooking | Warm the sun-dried tomato oil in the large saucepan over medium heat | Add the onion and a pinch of salt and cook, stirring, for 4–5 minutes | Add the celery and stir for 2 minutes | Add the garlic and stir for 1 minute | Add the sun-dried tomatoes and stir for 1 minute | Add the bell pepper chunks and stir for 2–3 minutes

Add the smoked paprika, thyme, cayenne pepper, and oregano to the pan and stir for 1 minute to coat | Add the jackfruit and stir gently for 3–4 minutes | Add the tomato paste and stir for 1 minute | Stir in the canned tomatoes | Add the water to the empty tomato can and add it to the pan | Add the bay leaf, reduce the heat to low, and simmer for 10 minutes, stirring occasionally

Now, make the finishing touches and serve | Take the sausages out of the oven and cut them into slices ¾ inch thick | Add the sausage slices and hot sauce to the pan and gently fold them into the jambalaya | Add the rice to the pan and fold it into the sauce | Thinly slice the scallions and add half of them to the pan | Squeeze in the lime juice and fold the juice and the scallions into the jambalaya | Taste and season to perfection with salt and lots of pepper | Plate up the jambalaya, garnish with the remaining scallions and the parsley, and serve

413 KCAL | LOW FAT | LOW SUGAR | FULL OF FIBER | PROTEIN PACKED

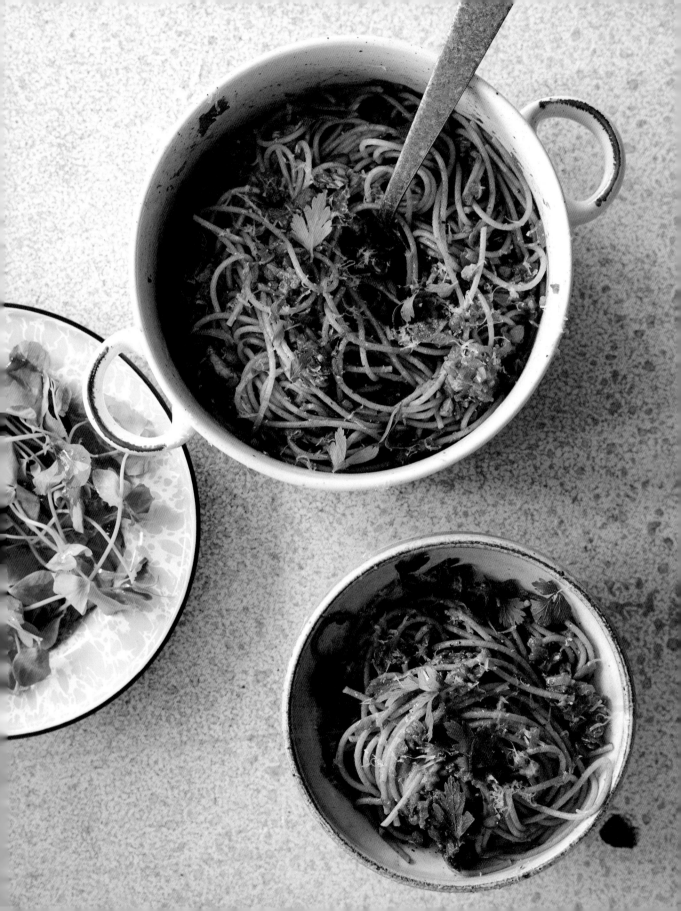

BANGIN' BOLOGNESE

One of our all-time favorite dishes is Bolognese. But, traditionally, it would be higher in saturated fat and served with lots of white pasta. Well, rejoice, because we've made a healthy version! First up, we're going for a higher ratio of sauce to pasta—and the sauce contains walnuts and lentils for a satisfying texture. We are also using whole wheat pasta, which is higher in fiber and much better for you.

SERVES 4

1 garlic clove
2 onions
1 (14 oz) can green lentils
¼ cup fresh thyme or 5 tsp dried thyme
⅓ cup walnuts
1 tbsp olive oil
1 (14 oz) can diced tomatoes
1 tbsp tomato paste
3 tbsp red wine
½ tsp chile flakes
1½ tsp dried oregano
1 tsp balsamic vinegar
½ tsp yeast extract (e.g., Marmite)
½ cup water
11 oz whole wheat spaghetti
salt and black pepper

TO SERVE

¾ oz vegan hard cheese, optional
½ cup fresh parsley leaves
7 oz salad greens

FINE GRATER OR MICROPLANE | FOOD PROCESSOR | LARGE SKILLET | LARGE SAUCEPAN | BOILING WATER

First, prep the ingredients | Peel and grate the garlic | Peel and finely chop the onions | Drain and rinse the lentils | Pick and roughly chop the thyme leaves—if you're using fresh rather than dried, set aside 1 teaspoon of the fresh leaves for garnishing | Blitz the walnuts in the food processor until coarsely ground

Now, make the lentil ragu | Heat the olive oil in the large skillet over medium heat | Add the onions and a pinch of salt and cook, stirring, for 4–5 minutes, until softened and translucent | Add the garlic and cook for another minute | Add the ground walnuts, lentils, canned tomatoes, tomato paste, red wine, chile flakes, oregano, thyme, balsamic vinegar, yeast extract, and water | Bring to a simmer and cook for 15–20 minutes, stirring regularly to prevent the sauce catching | It will look gray at first, but will darken as it cooks | Once the sauce has darkened in color and thickened considerably, taste and season to perfection with salt and pepper

While the ragu is simmering, cook your pasta | Put the saucepan on the burner | Pour the boiling water into the saucepan | Turn the heat right up | Sprinkle in a generous pinch of salt | Add the spaghetti and cook until al dente, following the instructions on the package | Remove ¼ cup of the starchy pasta cooking water and reserve | Drain the pasta in a colander | Add the cooked spaghetti and a splash of the pasta water to the ragu in the pan and stir in | Grate the hard cheese (if using) and chop the parsley leaves | Plate up the spaghetti and ragu, garnish with parsley (and thyme, if using fresh leaves) and serve immediately with green salad

492 KCAL | LOW SUGAR | FULL OF FIBER | PROTEIN PACKED

"CHORIZO" PASTA

Here we show you a clever way to make any veggie sausage taste just like chorizo. This dish is packed with protein, making it great for post exercise.

SERVES 4

PREHEAT OVEN TO 350°F | LINE A SHEET PAN WITH PARCHMENT PAPER | FINE GRATER OR MICROPLANE | 2 LARGE SAUCEPANS | BOILING WATER

FOR THE "CHORIZO"

6 vegan sausages
2–2½ tbsp olive oil
2 tsp smoked paprika
1 tsp ground fennel
1½ tsp cayenne pepper

FOR THE PASTA SAUCE

1 red onion
2 garlic cloves
2 red bell peppers
2 tbsp tomato paste
2 (14 oz) cans diced
    tomatoes
12 oz whole wheat
    penne pasta
6 oz fresh spinach leaves
salt and black pepper

TO GARNISH

1 lemon
½ cup fresh parsley
    leaves

First, prep the sausages and veggies | Put the sausages on the lined sheet pan, put the pan in the oven, and cook them for 20 minutes | Peel and finely dice the red onion | Peel and grate the garlic | Trim, halve, core, and thinly slice the bell peppers

Now, make the "chorizo" | Take the sausages out of the oven and cut them into rounds ⅓ inch thick | Heat 1 tablespoon of the olive oil in a large saucepan over medium-high heat | Add the pieces of sausage and fry, stirring gently, for 1 minute, until cooked on both sides (make sure you don't break them)—you may need a splash more oil | Sprinkle half the smoked paprika, half the ground fennel, and ½ teaspoon of the cayenne pepper into the pan | Cook the sausage pieces for 3–5 minutes, stirring, until crisped and fully coated in the spices | Transfer the pieces to a plate and set to one side | Clean out the pan with paper towels

Make the sauce in the same pan you cooked the "chorizo" in | Heat the remaining olive oil over medium heat | Add the red onion, sprinkle with a pinch of salt, and cook for 5–7 minutes | Add the garlic and stir for 1 minute | Add the red bell peppers and cook for 3 minutes | Sprinkle the remaining spices into the pan and stir for 30 seconds | Add the tomato paste and stir for 30 seconds | Tip the diced tomatoes into the pan | Half-fill one of the cans with water, pour into the pan, stir well, then reduce the heat and leave to simmer for 10–15 minutes, until thickened

While the sauce is simmering, cook the pasta | Put the second saucepan on the stove and pour in boiling water | Turn the heat right up | Sprinkle in a generous pinch of salt | Add the pasta to the pan and cook until al dente, following the instructions on the package

Taste the sauce and season to perfection with salt and pepper | Stir in the spinach | Drain the pasta, reserving a little of the cooking water | Pour the pasta into the tomato sauce and stir to completely coat, adding a little pasta water to loosen | Sprinkle the sausage pieces into the pan, fold them into the pasta for 1 minute | Halve the lemon | Serve immediately with a sprinkle of parsley and a squeeze of lemon juice

609 KCAL | LOW FAT | LOW SUGAR | FULL OF FIBER | PROTEIN PACKED

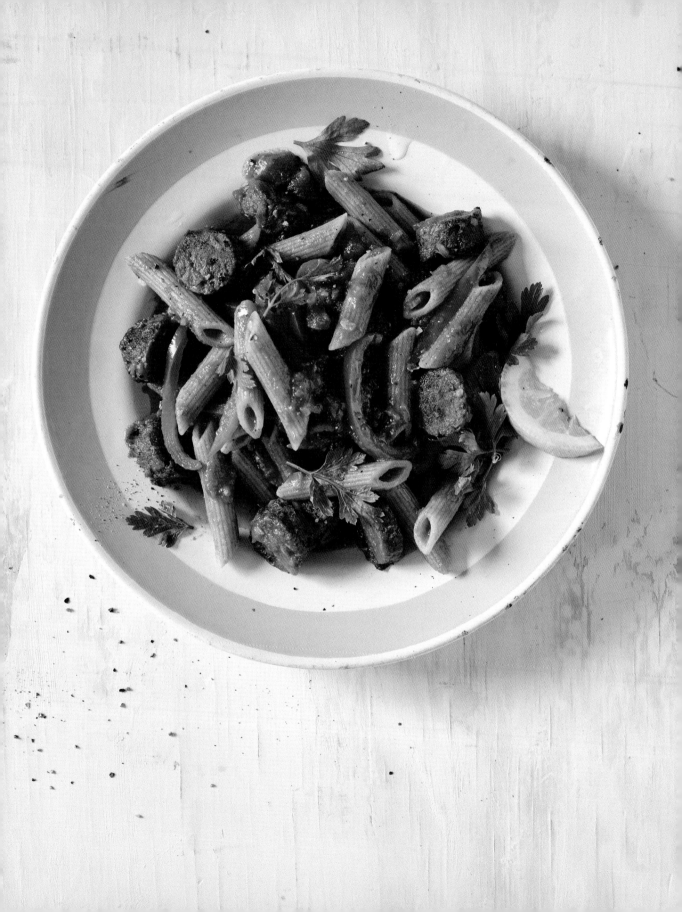

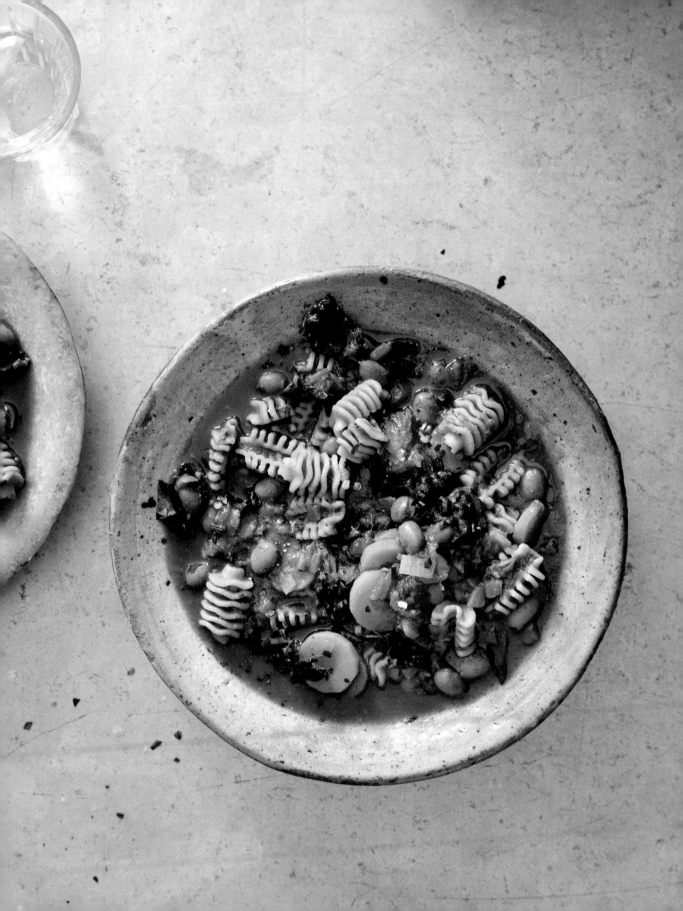

PASTA E FAGIOLI

Pasta e fagioli—literally, pasta and beans—is a hearty Italian dish, traditionally made using leftovers. We've used borlotti beans, which are high in fiber, protein, and folate, and kale to help you reach your daily greens goal. Treat this as a fridge-raid soup, adding whatever veggies you have to use up in your fridge.

SERVES 2

1 (14 oz) can borlotti or kidney beans

1 onion

4 garlic cloves

1 sprig fresh rosemary

6 sprigs fresh thyme

3½ oz kale

2 carrots

1 tbsp extra-virgin olive oil

7 tbsp red wine

1 (28 oz) can whole peeled tomatoes

1 bay leaf

½ tsp chile flakes, plus extra to serve

3½ oz whole wheat pasta, or broken tagliatelle

1 cup vegetable stock

1 cup water

salt and black pepper

FINE GRATER OR MICROPLANE | LARGE SAUCEPAN

First, prep the vegetables | Drain and rinse the beans | Peel and finely dice the onion | Peel and grate the garlic | Pick the rosemary and thyme leaves from the sprigs and roughly chop | Trim and discard the tough midribs from the kale, and thinly slice the leaves | Peel then slice the carrots into ⅛-inch-thick rounds

Now, cook the base of the dish | Heat the olive oil in the large saucepan over low heat | Add the onion and carrot and cook for 5 minutes, until softened slightly | Add the garlic, rosemary, and thyme and stir until fragrant | Add the red wine, increase the heat, and simmer for 3–4 minutes

Now, finish cooking the dish | Tip the canned tomatoes into the pan and break them up with a wooden spoon | Stir to combine, increase the heat to a simmer, and cook for 8–10 minutes, stirring every couple of minutes to prevent the mixture catching on the bottom of the pan | Add the beans, bay leaf, chile flakes, pasta, vegetable stock, and water and simmer for 10–12 minutes, until the pasta is cooked and the sauce is thick | Taste and season to perfection with salt and pepper, add the kale, and fold it into the sauce for 1 minute until well wilted

Time to serve! | Ladle the protein-packed pasta into two bowls, garnish with chile flakes, and serve immediately

526 KCAL | LOW FAT | LOW SUGAR | FULL OF FIBER | PROTEIN PACKED

BBQ SLOPPY JACKETS

We love giving junk food a healthy twist! This ragu is made from mushrooms and vegan crumbles and the stuffed sweet potatoes are served with a low-sugar BBQ sauce. It's high in protein so is the perfect gym food, and keeps you feeling fuller and satisfied for longer.

SERVES 2

2 medium sweet potatoes (about 10 oz each)

salt and black pepper

1 (1.4 oz) bag vegetable chips, to serve

3½ oz mixed salad greens, to serve

FOR THE SLOPPY JOE FILLING

5 oz mushrooms

1 red onion

2 garlic cloves

1 celery stalk

1 large carrot

1 tbsp olive oil, plus extra for the sweet potatoes

5 oz vegan crumbles

1 tsp mustard (e.g., yellow mustard)

¼ tsp hot sauce (e.g., Tabasco)

2½ tbsp BBQ sauce (low-sugar store-bought or use our BBQ Bourbon Sauce on page 169)

1 lime

¼ cup fresh parsley

PREHEAT OVEN TO 400°F | SHEET PAN | FOOD PROCESSOR | FINE GRATER OR MICROPLANE | LARGE SAUCEPAN

First, cook the sweet potatoes | Put the sweet potatoes on the sheet pan and pierce them a few times with a fork | Rub the potatoes with a splash of oil and scatter with a pinch of salt | Put the pan in the oven and bake the potatoes for 45–50 minutes, until the skin has started to crisp up and the flesh is tender

While the sweet potatoes are cooking, make the sloppy joe filling | Put the mushrooms in the food processor and blitz to finely mince | Peel and dice the red onion | Peel and grate the garlic | Trim and thinly slice the celery | Peel and grate the carrot

Heat the olive oil in the large saucepan over medium heat | Add the onion with a pinch of salt and cook, stirring, for 3–4 minutes | Add the garlic and stir for 1 minute | Add the celery and carrot and cook for 2–3 minutes | Add the mushrooms and vegan crumbles and cook for 8–10 minutes, stirring frequently, until the onion is soft and translucent and the mushroom and vegan crumbles have softened and browned slightly | Add the mustard and hot sauce and stir for 1 minute | Add the BBQ sauce and cook for another 4–5 minutes, then remove from the heat

Take the pan out of the oven | Leave the sweet potatoes to cool for 5 minutes | Carefully slice open the sweet potatoes and gently fluff the flesh with a fork | Spoon half the filling into each of the potatoes | Halve the lime and squeeze one half over each potato | Taste and season to perfection with salt and pepper, and garnish with parsley leaves | Serve immediately, with vegetable chips and a small side salad

668 KCAL | LOW FAT | LOW SUGAR | FULL OF FIBER | PROTEIN PACKED

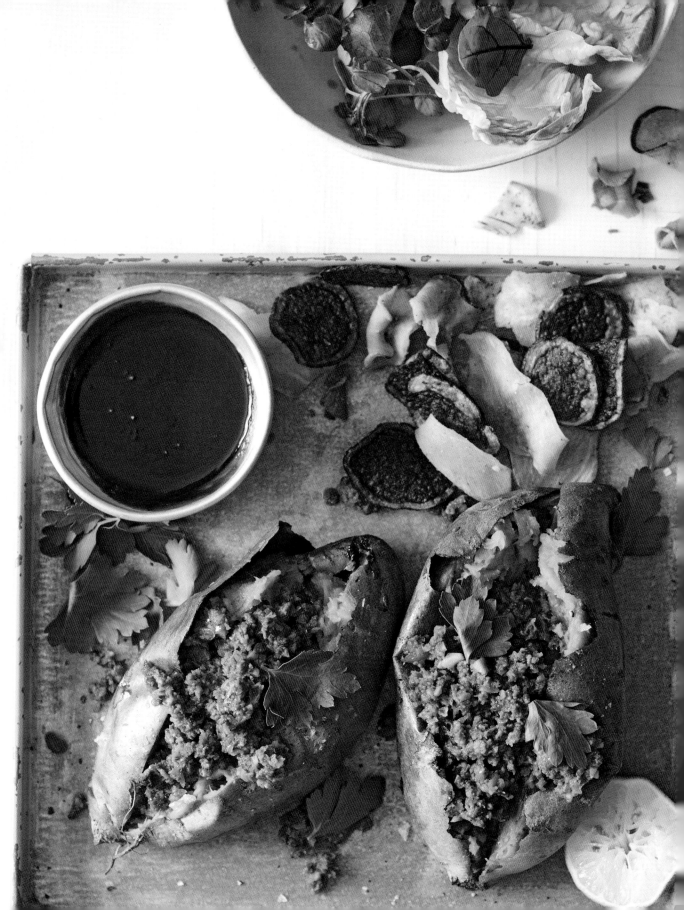

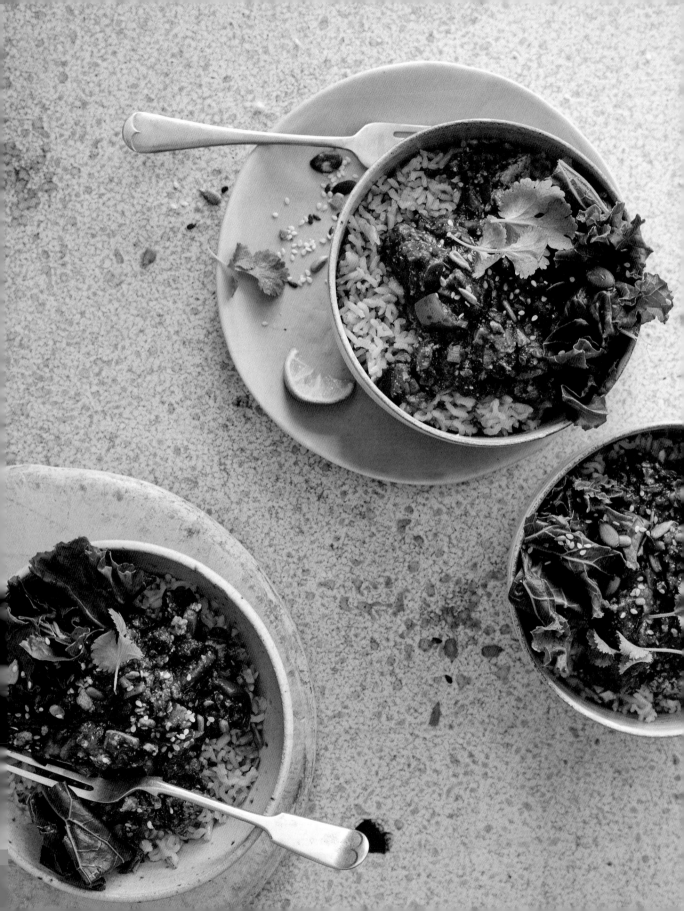

TOTAL PROTEIN CHILI

We created this chili for a presentation called "What Would We Eat on Mars?" Because, well, the first people on Mars would absolutely have to eat a vegan diet; they won't be rearing cows on the red planet! The chili is packed with protein and all the essential amino acids the body needs, and served with a big dose of health-giving kale.

SERVES 4

10oz firm tofu
1 red onion
2 garlic cloves
20 sprigs fresh cilantro
1 red bell pepper
⅓ cup sun-dried tomatoes
7 oz curly kale
1 tbsp olive oil, plus extra for drizzling
1 tsp chili powder (more to taste)
2 tsp ground cumin
2 tsp smoked paprika
1 tsp ground cinnamon
1 tsp dried oregano
2 (14 oz) cans diced tomatoes
1 tbsp balsamic vinegar
1 (14 oz) can black beans
1 vegetable bouillon cube
chile flakes, to taste
4 cups cooked basmati rice or 2 (8.8 oz) bags microwavable brown basmati rice
1 tbsp mixed seeds (such as pumpkin, sunflower, sesame, and flaxseed)
salt and black pepper
½ lime, to serve, optional

TOFU PRESS OR 2 CLEAN TEA TOWELS AND A WEIGHT SUCH AS A HEAVY BOOK | FINE GRATER OR MICROPLANE | LARGE SAUCEPAN | MEDIUM SAUCEPAN

First, press the tofu using a tofu press or place it between two clean tea towels, lay it on a plate, and put a weight on top | Leave for at least 30 minutes to drain off any liquid and firm up | Once the tofu has been pressed, crumble it into a bowl with your fingers and set aside

Meanwhile, prep your ingredients | Peel and finely chop the red onion | Peel and grate the garlic | Pick the cilantro leaves and thinly slice the stems | Trim, halve, and core the bell pepper, and cut it into bite-sized chunks | Finely chop the sun-dried tomatoes | Roughly chop the kale leaves

Heat the tablespoon of olive oil in the large saucepan over medium heat | Add the onion and a pinch of salt and cook, stirring, for 3–4 minutes | Add the garlic, cilantro stems, red pepper, and sun-dried tomatoes and cook for another 5 minutes | Add the crumbled tofu, chili powder, cumin, smoked paprika, cinnamon, and oregano and stir everything together well | Add the diced tomatoes, balsamic vinegar, and black beans (with the liquid from the can), crumble in the vegetable bouillon cube, and stir well | Reduce the heat to a gentle simmer and cook for 20–25 minutes, until thick

While the chili is nearly ready, cook the kale | Fill the medium saucepan with water, season well with salt, and bring to boil over high heat | Add the kale and blanch for 1–1½ minutes to soften | Drain the kale, pat it dry with paper towels, drizzle with a little olive oil, sprinkle with chile flakes, and set to one side

Remove the chili from the heat and stir in the cilantro leaves | Season to perfection with salt and pepper | Heat the rice, if necessary, or cook it following the package instructions | Plate up the rice, chili, and kale, sprinkle with the mixed seeds, and serve immediately with some lime to squeeze over the top if you like

557 KCAL | LOW SUGAR | FULL OF FIBER | PROTEIN PACKED

THAI NO-FISHCAKES

This might just be our favorite dish in the whole book. Remember that delicious, just-one-more dippiness of Thai fishcakes? Well we made them vegan-style, using jackfruit instead of fish, so you can still enjoy the gorgeously subtle spiciness of fishcakes with the freshness of the dipping sauce. Try it: it'll quickly become your favorite recipe, too.

SERVES 2

LARGE SAUCEPAN | POTATO MASHER | PREHEAT OVEN TO 425°F | SKILLET | LINE A SHEET PAN | SCISSORS

FOR THE JACKFRUIT FISHCAKES

2–3 medium potatoes (about 1 lb)

3 scallions

1½-inch piece fresh ginger (about ½ oz)

1 nori sheet, optional

1 (14 oz) can young green jackfruit in water

10 sprigs fresh cilantro

1 tbsp olive oil

2 tbsp vegan Thai red curry paste

1 tsp soy sauce, plus extra to taste

salt and black pepper

FOR THE THAI-TARE SAUCE

1 lime

½ oz fresh ginger

1 tsp vegan Thai red curry paste

1 tsp soy sauce

TO SERVE

1 lime

½ small fresh red chile

3½ oz mixed salad greens

First, prep the potatoes | Peel then cut them into 1-inch chunks and put them in the large pan of cold salted water | Put the pan over high heat, bring to a boil, and cook for 8–12 minutes, until tender | Drain the potatoes, tip into a large bowl, and mash with a potato masher

Trim and thinly slice the scallions | Peel the ginger by scraping off the skin with a spoon, then grate | Snip the nori sheet (if using) with scissors into small pieces | Drain the jackfruit, rinse under a cold tap, and pat dry with a clean tea towel or paper towels | Pull the jackfruit into pieces with two forks, so it resembles flaked tuna | Separate the cilantro leaves and stems and chop the stems

Now, make the fishcakes | Put the skillet over medium heat and add the oil | Add the scallions and ginger and sauté for a couple of minutes, then add the jackfruit, cilantro stems, and nori (if using) | Sauté for another 5 minutes, stirring often, then add the red curry paste and soy sauce | Reduce the heat to low and cook for 10 minutes, stirring often | When the jackfruit is lightly browned and tastes fantastic, add the mashed potato, mix well, and fry for another 5 minutes, until the potato has browned slightly | Remove from the heat, taste, and season to perfection with salt, pepper, and a splash more soy sauce

Leave until cool enough to handle, then use your hands to form the mixture into 6 even-sized patties | Place them on the lined sheet pan, put in the oven, and bake for 17–20 minutes, until lightly browned

While the fishcakes are baking, make the Thai-tare sauce | Halve the lime and squeeze the juice | Finely chop the reserved cilantro leaves | Peel the ginger by scraping off the skin with a spoon, then grate | Put all the ingredients in a bowl and mix to form a paste | Add water if required, to get a dippable, quite loose consistency

Cut the whole lime into wedges and chop the chile | Serve the fishcakes with the sauce, a small mixed salad, and lime wedges

442 KCAL | LOW FAT | LOW SUGAR | FULL OF FIBER

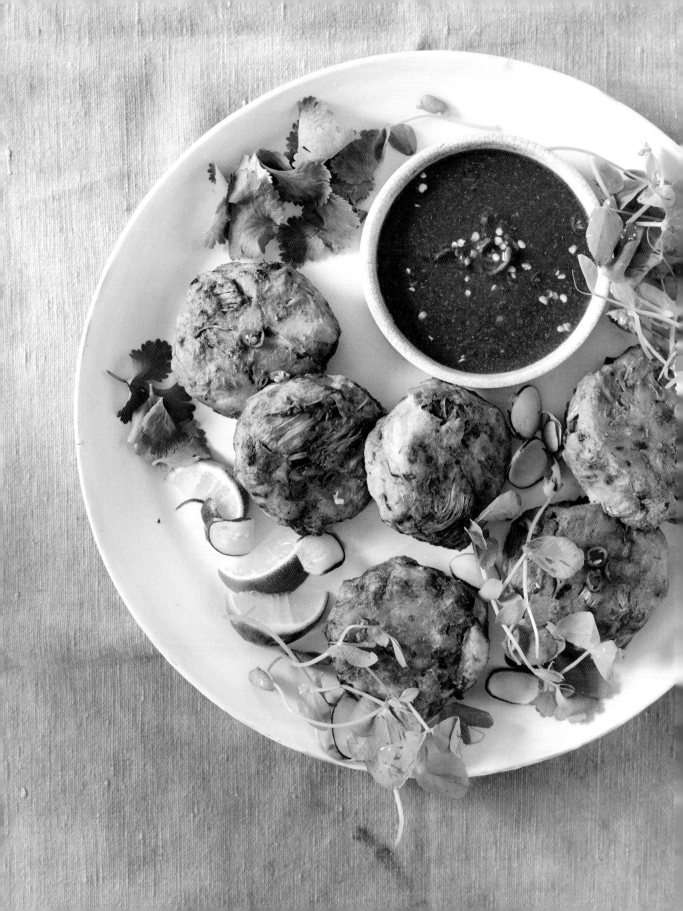

GOAN-STYLE CURRY

This hot, satisfying curry is bursting with all the sweet spiciness of South Indian cooking. We use banana blossom and mixed mushrooms to provide a great fishy texture, but you can double up the mushrooms if you prefer.

SERVES 4

2 LARGE SAUCEPANS | FINE GRATER OR MICROPLANE | PESTLE AND MORTAR

First, make the curry base | Peel and thinly slice the shallots | Rip the stem from the chile and finely chop | Place one of the saucepans over medium heat and add the canola oil | Add the shallots, green chile, and a pinch of salt to the pan and cook, stirring regularly, for 4–5 minutes, until softened | Take the pan off the heat

Now, make the curry paste | Warm the second saucepan over medium heat, add the mustard and cumin seeds, and toast until fragrant | Tip the seeds into the mortar and grind them with the pestle to a powder | Add the ground coriander, cayenne pepper, paprika, turmeric, chile flakes, and curry leaves and grind to a coarse powder | Peel and grate the garlic | Peel the ginger by scraping off the skin with a spoon, then grate | Add the garlic, ginger, and soy sauce to the mortar and mix to form a paste | Taste and season to perfection with salt and pepper

Marinate the banana blossom | Drain and rinse the banana blossom and pat it dry with paper towels | Shred the banana blossom into bite-sized pieces | Put 2 teaspoons of the tamarind paste and a pinch of salt in a mixing bowl, add the banana blossom, toss to combine, and leave to marinate for 10 minutes

Make the curry | Roughly chop the tomatoes | Put the pan containing the shallots and chile back over medium heat, add the curry paste, and stir for 2 minutes, until fragrant | Add the tomatoes and cook, stirring, for 3–4 minutes | Add the coconut milk, vegetable stock, remaining tamarind paste, and maple syrup and simmer for 10 minutes, until the liquid has reduced

Cut the mushrooms into bite-sized pieces | Trim and halve the green beans | Add the mushrooms, green beans, and banana blossom to the curry and simmer for 7–8 minutes, until cooked through

Time to serve! | While the curry is simmering, cut the limes into wedges | Heat the rice, if necessary, or cook it following the package instructions, then add the rice to serving bowls | Serve the curry over the rice, garnish with cilantro leaves, and serve with lime wedges

FOR THE CURRY PASTE

- ½ tsp black mustard seeds
- 1 tsp cumin seeds
- 1 tsp ground coriander
- ½ tsp cayenne pepper
- ½ tsp smoked paprika
- ½ tsp ground turmeric
- ½ tbsp chile flakes
- 10 dried curry leaves
- 3 garlic cloves
- 1¼-inch piece fresh ginger
- 1 tsp soy sauce
- salt and black pepper

FOR THE CURRY

- 2 echalions (banana shallots)
- 1 fresh green chile
- 1 tbsp canola oil
- 1 (18 oz) can banana blossom in brine
- 3 tsp tamarind paste
- 12 cherry tomatoes
- 1¼ cups reduced-fat coconut milk
- 1⅔ cups vegetable stock
- 1 tsp maple syrup
- 7 oz mixed mushrooms
- 3½ oz green beans
- 2 limes
- 4 cups cooked basmati rice or 2 (8.8 oz) bags microwavable brown basmati rice
- ¼ cup fresh cilantro leaves, to serve

330 KCAL | LOW FAT | LOW SUGAR | FULL OF FIBER

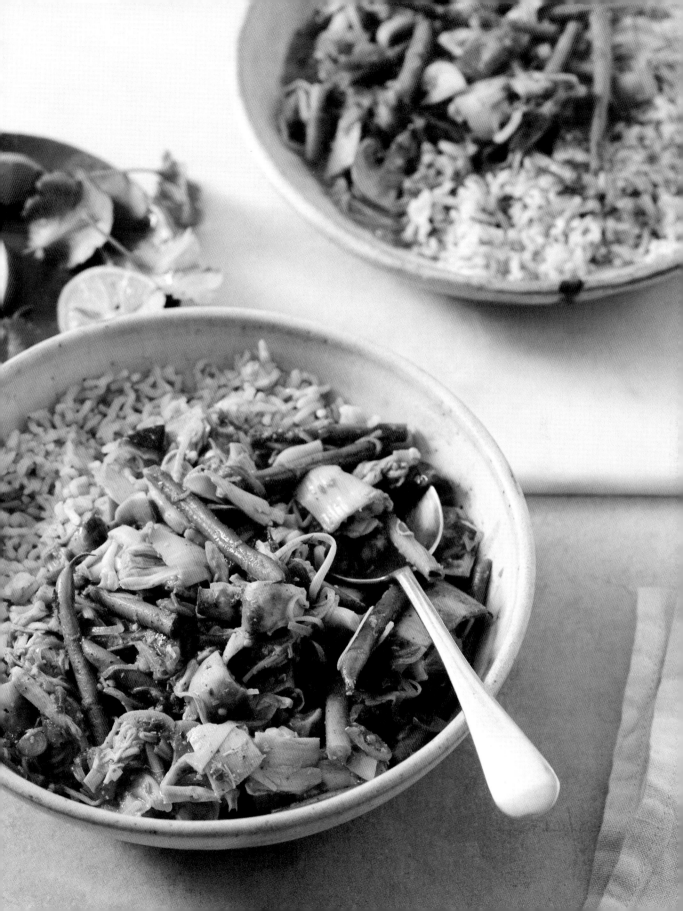

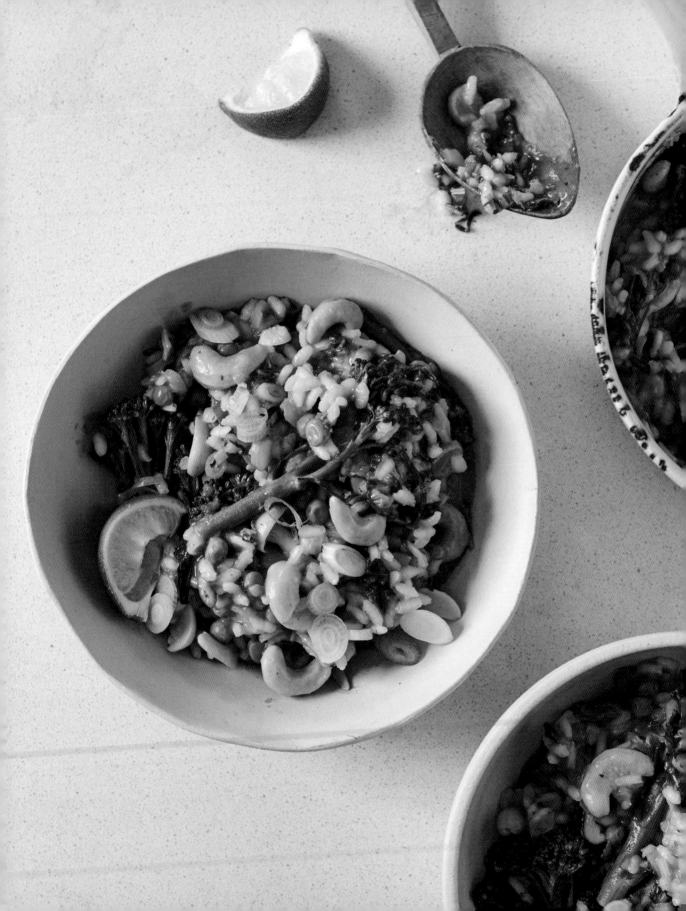

ASIAN-STYLE RISOTTO

We decided to take risotto on a little bit of a world tour! Cooked much like a traditional risotto, we've used Asian flavors and vegetables to make it spicy, peppery, and deliciously complex. Taste and adjust your seasoning so the spice levels are where you want them – and feel free to use a bit of hot sauce at the end to up the fire.

SERVES 4

8 scallions
2 large garlic cloves
2-inch piece fresh ginger
1 fresh green chile
⅓ cup cashews
30 sprigs fresh cilantro
   (about 1 oz)
7 oz shiitake mushrooms
7 oz bok choy
2 cups vegetable stock
   mixed with 2 cups
   water
7 oz broccolini
1 lime
1 tbsp olive oil
1 tbsp sesame oil
2 tbsp white miso paste
generous 1 cup risotto
   rice
¾ cup frozen peas or
   shelled edamame
1 tbsp soy sauce,
   or to taste
salt and black pepper

FINE GRATER OR MICROPLANE | MEDIUM SAUCEPAN | LARGE SOUP POT

First, prep your ingredients | Trim and thinly slice the scallions | Peel and grate the garlic | Peel the ginger by scraping off the skin with a spoon, then grate it | Rip the stem from the chile, cut it in half lengthwise, and remove the seeds (if you like), then finely chop | Roughly chop the cashews | Pick the cilantro leaves and finely chop the stems | Roughly chop the shiitake mushrooms | Trim and finely dice the white part of the bok choy and roughly shred the green part | Heat the stock and water in the medium saucepan and keep over low heat | Trim and finely dice the broccolini stalks, keeping the florets whole | Cut the lime into wedges

Warm both the oils over medium heat in the large soup pot | Add three-quarters of the scallions, the garlic, ginger, chile, and cilantro stems and cook, stirring, for 2 minutes | Add the diced cashews and white miso paste and stir for 1 minute | Add the shiitake mushrooms and stir for 2 minutes | Add the white shreds of bok choy and stir for 1 minute | Add the risotto rice and stir for 1 minute

Add ¾ cup of the hot stock to the soup pot and stir concanuously until all the liquid has been absorbed | Repeat this process three more times until you're left with about ¾ cup stock | Add the stalks of the broccolini after the rice has been cooking for 10 minutes | Add the remaining bok choy, peas or edamame, and broccolini florets and fold them into the risotto for 30 seconds | Add the remaining stock and the soy sauce and stir until the liquid has been absorbed and the risotto has a creamy consistency | The rice should take about 20 minutes to cook–the grains should be tender but still with a little bite

Add half of the cilantro leaves and half the remaining scallions to the risotto and fold them in | Taste the risotto and season to perfection with salt and pepper (and more soy sauce if you wish) | Plate up the risotto, top with the remaining cilantro leaves and scallions, and serve immediately, with lime wedges

442 KCAL | LOW FAT | LOW SUGAR | FULL OF FIBER | PROTEIN PACKED

CAT'S CURRYFLOWER

Cathy is a fully-fledged member of team BOSH! and responsible for most of the food videos on our channels. She loved our Buffalo cauliflower wings so much that she asked us to create a curry-flavored version just for her. So here it is: a hot and spicy cauliflower dish to tuck in to or nibble on. It also makes a perfect side for any spicy feast or party snack.

SERVES 2

1 medium head cauliflower
1 tbsp olive oil
2 cups cooked basmati rice or 1 (8.8 oz) bag microwavable brown basmati rice
1 scallion
1 small Little Gem lettuce
½ lime
1 tsp white sesame seeds
salt

FOR THE SPICE PASTE

2 tbsp plus 1 tsp red miso paste
1½ tbsp maple syrup
½ tsp cayenne pepper
½ tsp smoked paprika
1½ tbsp water
2 tsp vegetable oil

PREHEAT OVEN TO 400°F | SHEET PAN

First, prep the cauliflower | Break the cauliflower into florets, put the florets in a mixing bowl, drizzle with the olive oil, sprinkle with a little salt, and toss to coat | Tip the cauliflower florets onto the sheet pan, put the pan in the oven, and roast the florets for 10 minutes

Now, make the spice paste | In the same mixing bowl, add the red miso paste, maple syrup, cayenne pepper, and smoked paprika and stir to combine | Stir in water and oil to loosen the paste

Coat the cauliflower florets | Take the roasted cauliflower florets out of the oven and pour over the spice paste | Toss well, making sure the florets are well coated | Return the pan to the oven and roast for another 15 minutes

Prep and plate up the dish | Heat the rice, if necessary, or cook it following the package instructions | Trim and thinly slice the scallion | Trim and thinly slice the lettuce | Cut the half lime into wedges | Take the cauliflower out of the oven | Plate up the rice, cauliflower, and lettuce | Sprinkle with the sesame seeds and scallion and serve with the lime wedges

347 KCAL | LOW SUGAR | FULL OF FIBER

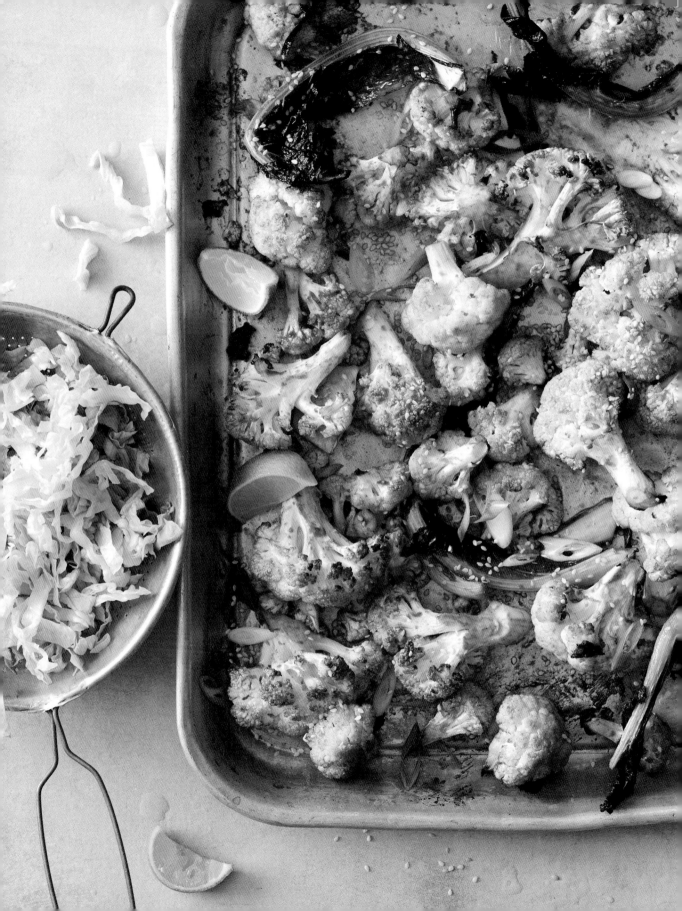

EMJ'S HEARTY HOTPOT

EmJ is Henry's fiancée and she loves a warming, hearty hotpot! In fact, most things she cooks end up being some sort of hotpot. Once she made a hotpot lasagna, which may one day make it on to our channel as a recipe. Anyway, this is her ultimate hotpot—easy to make, packed with hearty flavors. If you want to jazz this up even more, serve with a bit of toasted pita and some hummus.

SERVES 4

1 red bell pepper
1 yellow bell pepper
1 tsp smoked paprika
6 vegan sausages
1 red onion
3 garlic cloves
2 sprigs fresh rosemary
6 sprigs fresh thyme
1 (14 oz) can cannellini beans
½ tbsp olive oil, plus extra for drizzling
½ tsp chile flakes
½ tbsp balsamic vinegar
2 tbsp tomato paste
1 cup red wine
2 (14 oz) cans cherry tomatoes
½ cup vegetable stock
½ tsp yeast extract (e.g., Marmite)
1 tsp Henderson's Relish or vegan Worcestershire sauce, optional
3½ oz kale
salt and black pepper

PREHEAT OVEN TO 350°F | LINE A LARGE SHEET PAN WITH PARCHMENT PAPER | FINE GRATER OR MICROPLANE | SOUP POT

....

Trim, halve, and core the bell peppers, then cut them into bite-sized chunks | Put the peppers and smoked paprika in a mixing bowl, add a drizzle of olive oil and some salt and pepper, and mix to coat | Tip the peppers onto the lined sheet pan | Add the vegan sausages to the pan, put the pan in the oven, and roast for 20–25 minutes

Peel and finely dice the red onion | Peel and grate the garlic | Pick the rosemary and thyme leaves from the sprigs and finely chop them | Drain and rinse the cannellini beans

Heat the olive oil in the soup pot over medium heat | Add the red onion and a pinch of salt and cook, stirring, for 2 minutes | Add the garlic, chile flakes, and diced rosemary and thyme and cook for 1 minute | Add the balsamic vinegar and tomato paste and stir for 1 minute to combine | Add the red wine and simmer for 3 minutes, then add the cannellini beans and canned tomatoes | Split the stock evenly between the empty cans then tip the stock from the cans into the soup pot and add the yeast extract and Henderson's Relish or Worcestershire sauce (if using) | Let the hotpot simmer for 10 minutes, stirring often to prevent it catching on the bottom of the pan

Take the sausages and peppers out of the oven | Cut the sausages into rounds ⅓ inch thick, then add the sausages and peppers to the pot, stir to combine, and simmer for another 5 minutes, stirring frequently

Remove the tough midribs from the kale and thinly slice the leaves | Add the kale to the pot and simmer for another 3 minutes | Taste the hotpot and season to perfection with salt and pepper | Spoon the hotpot into bowls and serve immediately

343 KCAL | LOW FAT | LOW SUGAR | FULL OF FIBER | PROTEIN PACKED

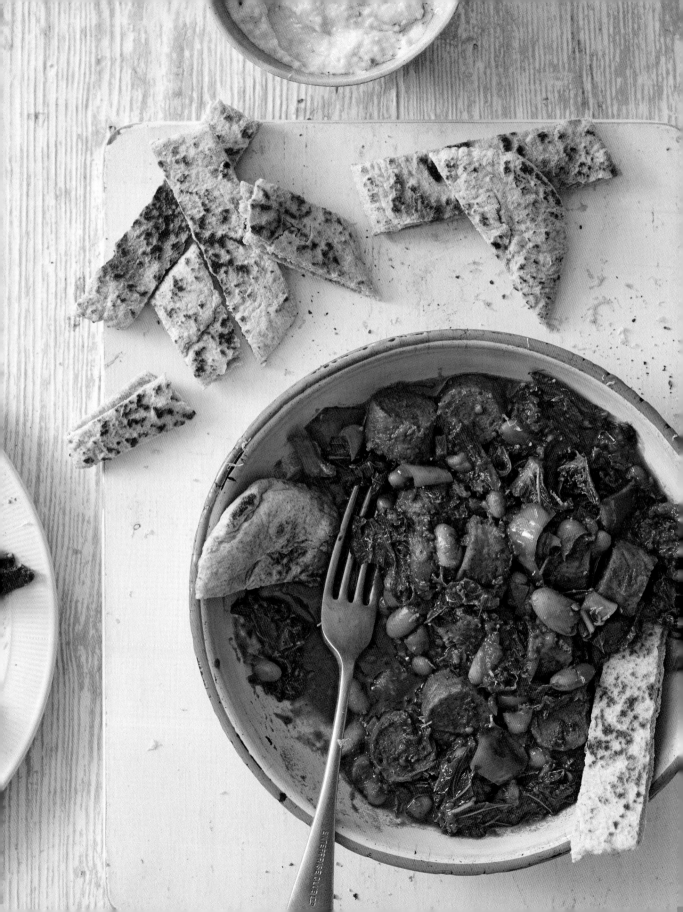

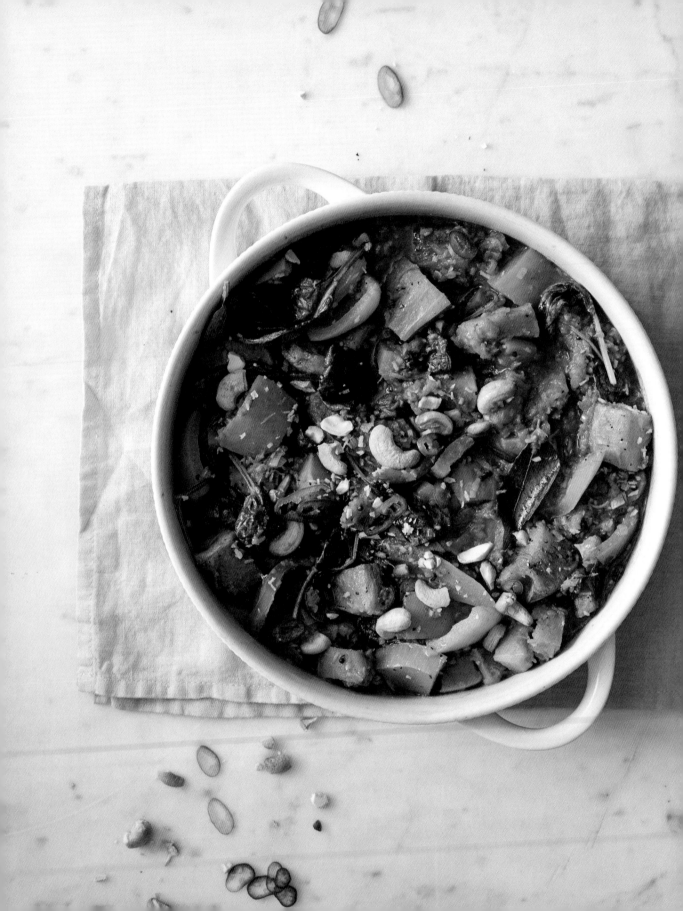

SUNNY SRI LANKAN CURRY

A big, rich Sri Lankan curry is one of our favorite dishes, but typically they are super high in saturated fat due to the coconut milk. We've tempered this bad boy down, using reduced-fat coconut milk and some water and shredded coconut instead, but it's still big on flavor. Serve it on its own, or if you're feeling extra hungry, add a portion of brown basmati rice.

SERVES 4

- 1 small butternut squash (about 14 oz)
- 1 tsp vegetable oil
- 2½ tbsp cashews
- 2 echalions (banana shallots)
- 3 large garlic cloves
- 2-inch piece fresh ginger (about ¾ oz)
- 1 fresh green bird's-eye chile
- 1 red bell pepper
- 1 orange bell pepper
- 1 tsp coconut oil
- 1 tsp ground turmeric
- 1 tbsp curry powder
- 1 tbsp black mustard seeds
- 1 tbsp tomato paste
- 15 curry leaves, optional
- ¾ cup reduced-fat coconut milk
- ¾ cup water
- 2 tbsp unsweetened shredded coconut
- 3½ oz baby spinach
- ½ lime
- ¼ cup fresh cilantro leaves, optional
- salt and black pepper

PREHEAT OVEN TO 350°F | LINE A SHEET PAN WITH PARCHMENT PAPER | SMALL SHEET PAN | FINE GRATER OR MICROPLANE | LARGE SAUCEPAN OR WOK

First, prep the squash and cashews | Trim and peel the butternut squash, halve it, and scoop out the seeds | Cut the squash into 1-inch cubes | Spread the cubes over the lined sheet pan, drizzle over the vegetable oil, season with salt and pepper, put the pan in the oven, and roast for 30 minutes, until tender | Toast the cashews in the oven on the small sheet pan for the last 5–8 minutes, until golden, then roughly chop

Now, prep the rest of your ingredients | Peel and finely dice the shallots | Peel and grate the garlic | Peel the ginger by scraping off the skin with a spoon, then grate | Rip the stem from the chile, cut it in half lengthwise, and remove the seeds if you prefer, then finely slice | Trim, halve, core, and dice the bell peppers

Time to cook the curry! | Heat the coconut oil in the large saucepan or wok over medium heat | Add the shallots and a pinch of salt and cook, stirring, for 4–5 minutes | Add the garlic, ginger, and chile and stir for 1 minute | Add the turmeric, curry powder, mustard seeds, tomato paste, and curry leaves (if using) and stir for 30 seconds | Add the peppers and stir for 1 minute | Pour the coconut milk, water, and half the shredded coconut into the pan (reserve the rest to sprinkle over the curry at the end) | Stir to combine, turn up the heat, and simmer for 4–5 minutes

Add the spinach and stir to wilt | Add the roasted butternut squash cubes and fold them into the curry | Squeeze the juice from the lime into the pan and fold it into the sauce

Taste the curry, season to perfection with salt and pepper, sprinkle with the cashews, cilantro leaves (if using), and remaining shredded coconut, and serve immediately

213 KCAL | LOW FAT | LOW SUGAR | FULL OF FIBER | PROTEIN PACKED

SALAD LASAGNA

Nothing beats a comforting plate of lasagna. This healthy version is packed with greens including fava beans, asparagus, and peas, as well as nutritional yeast, which is a real nutrient bomb. But most important, this dish is easy to make and absolutely delicious. We precook the pasta sheets so they cook more quickly in the oven, and we use a touch of dairy-free cheese to round things off.

SERVES 4

6 scallions
6 garlic cloves
1 lb asparagus
1½ oz fresh mint sprigs
3½ oz kale
1 lemon
2½ oz dairy-free cheese
9 oz lasagna sheets
2 tsp olive oil, plus extra
   for frying
2¼ cups frozen peas
2⅓ cups frozen fava
   beans
salad greens, to serve

FOR THE BÉCHAMEL

2 tablespoons olive oil
6 tbsp all-purpose flour
¼ cup nutritional yeast
2½ cups unsweetened
   plant-based milk
salt and black pepper

FINE GRATER OR MICROPLANE | BOILING WATER | 2 LARGE SAUCEPANS | LARGE, DEEP SKILLET | 9-INCH SQUARE LASAGNA DISH

First, prep the vegetables | Trim and thinly slice the scallions | Peel and grate the garlic | Cut the tips off the asparagus spears, then trim and thinly slice the stalks | Pick the mint leaves from the stems and roughly chop | Remove the tough midribs from the kale and roughly chop the leaves | Zest and halve the lemon | Grate the dairy-free cheese

Now, prep the lasagna sheets | Add 1 teaspoon of olive oil to a large pan filled with boiling water (this is essential to stop the pasta sticking as it cooks) | Add the lasagna sheets to the water and cook for 6-8 minutes over medium heat until al dente, moving frequently with tongs to ensure the sheets don't stick | Using tongs, carefully transfer the lasagna sheets one by one to a separate pan of cold water with another teaspoon of oil–this will help ensure the pasta doesn't stick together

Now, prep the filling | Warm a drizzle of olive oil in the large, deep skillet over high heat, add the scallions, and cook, stirring, for 1 minute | Add the garlic and stir for 1 minute until aromatic | Add the asparagus stalks, peas, and fava beans and stir for 1 minute | Add the kale and stir for 1 minute | Add the mint, lemon zest, and the juice from half the lemon and stir for 3-5 minutes, until the kale has wilted and the beans are cooked through | Transfer the vegetables to a dish and set to one side

recipe continued . . .

520 KCAL | LOW SUGAR | FULL OF FIBER | PROTEIN PACKED

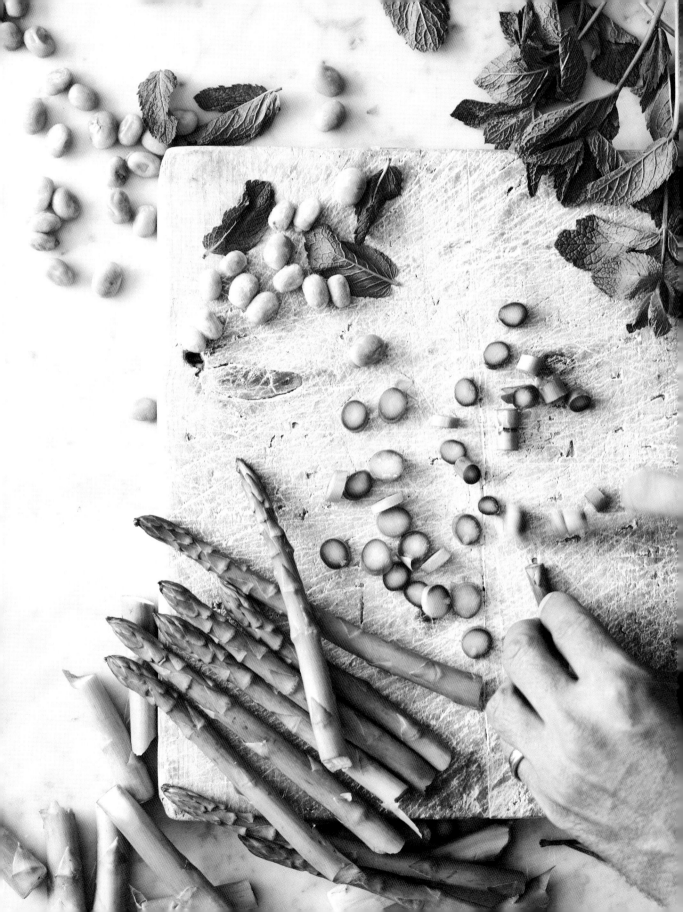

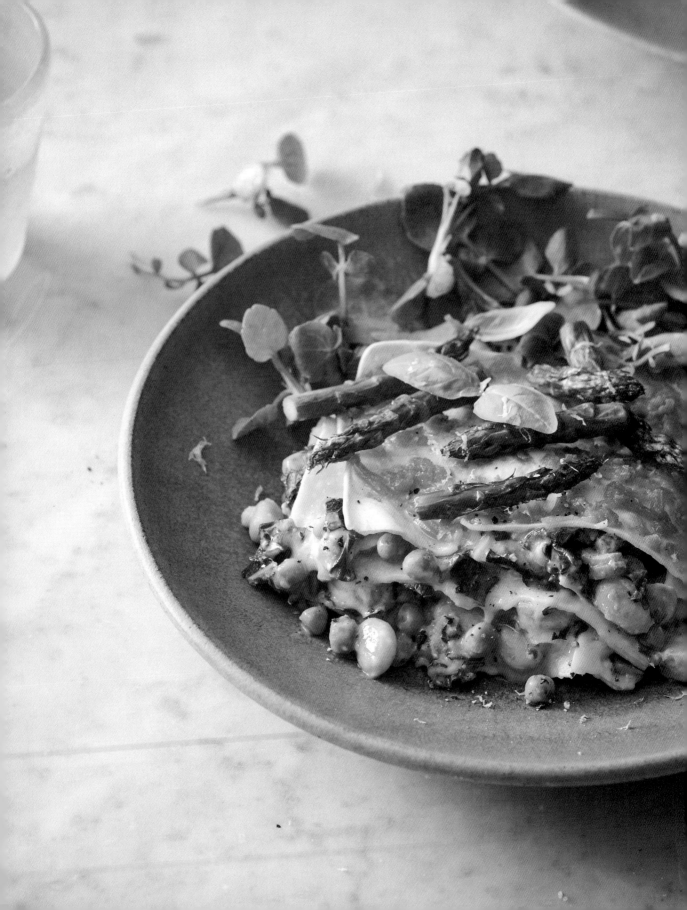

. . . continued from previous page

Make the béchamel | Put the empty pan back on the burner and warm the olive oil over medium heat | Add the flour and nutritional yeast and stir for 1 minute to combine | Gradually pour the milk into the pan and stir concanuously until the béchamel has thickened and has reached the consistency of double cream

Add the dish of vegetables to the pan and fold them into the béchamel | Taste the sauce and season to perfection with salt and pepper

Now, layer your lasagna | Add a quarter of the vegetable mixture to the lasagna dish and spread it out evenly | Remove the lasagna sheets from the water one by one with tongs, using the sheets to cover the vegetable mixture | Repeat this process until no more ingredients remain, finishing with a layer of lasagna sheets | Sprinkle a generous helping of grated dairy-free cheese all over the top of the lasagna | Top with the asparagus tips | Put the lasagna under the broiler for 5–7 minutes on medium-high heat, until tiny brown spots appear and it begins to crisp around the edges—be careful not to let the top of the lasagna burn

Time to serve | Remove the lasagna from the broiler and cut it into slices | Plate up the slices and serve with a simple green salad

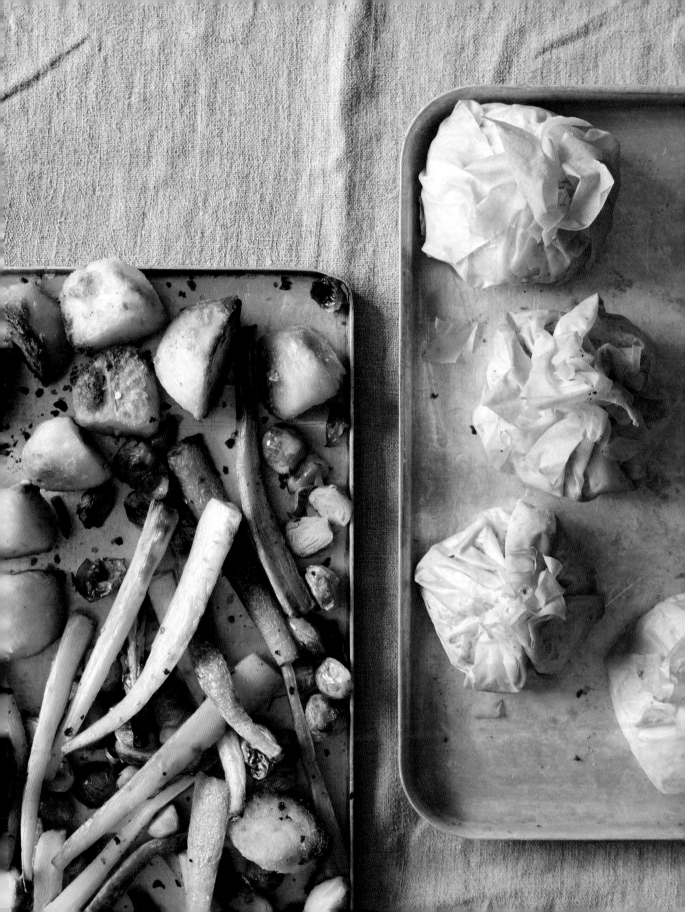

EASY & HEALTHY ROAST DINNER

We decided to give the BOSH! classic Mushroom Wellington from our first book a healthy makeover, using light phyllo pastry sheets to wrap delicious little mushroom parcels. Combine it with our hearty-yet-light gravy for your next Sunday roast.

SERVES 4

FOR THE ROAST VEGGIES

6 medium russet potatoes (about 2¼ lb)

3 medium carrots (about 10 oz)

3 medium parsnips (about 10 oz)

5 oz Brussels sprouts

1 tbsp olive oil

salt and black pepper

FOR THE RICH GRAVY

2 small red onions

2 garlic cloves

1 tbsp olive oil

1 tbsp cornstarch

2 tbsp water

1 tbsp tomato paste

1 tsp yeast extract (e.g., Marmite)

1 tsp maple syrup

1¼ cups red wine

1½ cups vegetable stock

salt and black pepper

ingredients list and recipe continued on next page . . .

PREHEAT OVEN TO 350°F | 2 LARGE SHEET PANS | 1 LARGE SAUCEPAN | FINE GRATER OR MICROPLANE | 1 MEDIUM SAUCEPAN | FOOD PROCESSOR | LARGE SKILLET

First, prep the roast vegetables | Peel and quarter the potatoes | Peel the carrots and parsnips and cut them into small, similar-sized batons | Trim and halve the Brussels sprouts

Place the potatoes and a pinch of salt in the large saucepan, cover with cold water, put the pan over high heat, bring to a boil, and simmer for 6–7 minutes, until slightly tender | Drain the potatoes, return them to the pan, and let them steam-dry for 2–3 minutes, shaking the pan gently to fluff the edges | Put the olive oil and a pinch each of salt and pepper in a large bowl | Add the potatoes, carrots, and parsnips and toss to coat | Take the potatoes out of the bowl, place them on one of the sheet pans and put the pan to one side | Add the Brussels sprouts to the bowl with the carrots and parsnips and toss to coat

Now, make the gravy | Peel and thinly slice the red onions | Peel and grate the garlic | Heat the olive oil in the medium saucepan over medium heat | Add the onion and a small pinch of salt and cook, stirring, for 5–6 minutes | Add the garlic and stir for 1 minute | Combine the cornstarch with the water in a cup and stir to make a slurry | Add the slurry to the pan along with the tomato paste, yeast extract, and maple syrup and stir to combine | Add the red wine and cook, stirring, for 3–4 minutes | Add the vegetable stock, stir, increase the heat, and simmer for 10–15 minutes to thicken, stirring occasionally to prevent the gravy catching on the bottom of the pan | Taste, season to perfection with salt and pepper, and set the pan to one side (If you prefer a smooth gravy, pass it through a sieve)

While the gravy is thickening, prep the mushrooms | Peel and grate the largest of the 3 garlic cloves into a bowl | Add a pinch each of salt and pepper and a drizzle of olive oil and stir | Place the 4 large mushrooms on the second sheet pan gill side up | Rub the garlic paste into the gills of the mushrooms | Put the mushrooms in the oven and bake for 10–12 minutes | Remove the pan from the oven and set the mushrooms to one side

881 KCAL | LOW FAT | LOW SUGAR | FULL OF FIBER

. . . continued from previous page

FOR THE WELLINGTON PHYLLO PARCELS

3 garlic cloves

2 tsp olive oil

4 large cremini mushrooms or small portobello mushrooms, plus 5 oz cremini mushrooms for the filling

1 small red onion

2 sprigs fresh rosemary

3 sprigs fresh thyme

3 oz vacuum-packed cooked chestnuts

½ cup pecans

1 slice whole wheat bread (about 1¾ oz)

2 tbsp white wine

4 sheets vegan phyllo pastry

cooking oil spray

salt and black pepper

While the mushrooms are cooking, prep the first part of your Wellington filling | Peel and halve the red onion | Peel the remaining 2 garlic cloves | Put the red onion, garlic, and 5 oz cremini mushrooms in the food processor and blitz into a fine mince | Transfer to a bowl and put to one side | Remove the leaves from the rosemary and thyme and finely chop | Put the chestnuts, pecans, and whole wheat bread in the food processor and blitz to form a textured filling

Now, start the roasting process | Put the pan of potatoes in the oven and roast for 40 minutes

Carry on building the Wellington parcels | Warm the remaining teaspoon of olive oil in the skillet over medium heat | If the onion and mushroom mixture has released liquid, drain it briefly in a sieve | Add the mixture to the pan with a pinch of salt and cook, stirring, for 4–5 minutes | Add the finely diced rosemary and thyme and stir for 1 minute | Add the white wine and stir for 3–4 minutes | Take the pan off the heat | Add the chestnut, pecan, and bread mixture and fold it into the rest of the ingredients to form a thick ball of filling | Taste and season to perfection with salt and pepper

Now, continue the roasting process | Take the pan out of the oven, turn the potatoes, and put the carrot and parsnips on the pan | Put the pan back in the oven for 20 minutes

Build your Wellington parcels | Cut the phyllo pastry sheets in half so you have 8 squares | Lay the sheets out in piles of two, arranged so the two sheets are overlapping at different angles to create star shapes | Divide the filling into 8 equal pieces, roll one of the pieces into a ball, place one ball in the center of a pastry star and press it to form a ⅓-inch-thick disc | Take one of the roasted mushrooms and place it in the center of the disc | Take another piece of the filling, roll it into a ball, and flatten it out into a ⅓-inch-thick disk between your hands | Place the disc of filling on top of the mushroom and mold the two pieces of filling around the mushroom to form a ball, ensuring the edges are sealed | Pull the exposed sheets of phyllo pastry up around the ball and twist the tops together so the Wellington pastry parcel is tightly wrapped, being careful not to rip the pastry | Spray the tops of the pastry parcels with a little cooking spray | Repeat this process with the remaining ingredients to make four Wellington parcels

Now, complete the roasting process | Take the pan of potatoes, parsnips, and carrots out of the oven and add the Brussels sprouts to the pan | Put the Wellington phyllo parcels on a separate pan and put the pans back in the oven for 20 minutes, until all the vegetables are well roasted and the parcels are golden and crispy

Prepare to serve your dinner | Warm the gravy through so it's hot and gently steaming | Remove the pans from the oven, plate up the Wellington parcels and roasted vegetables, pour over the gravy, and serve immediately

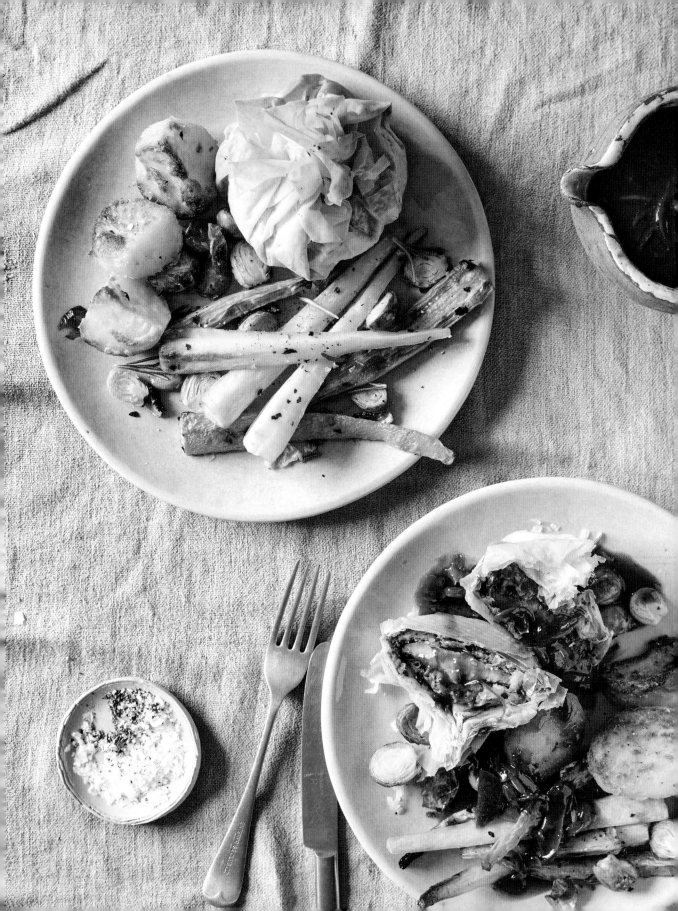

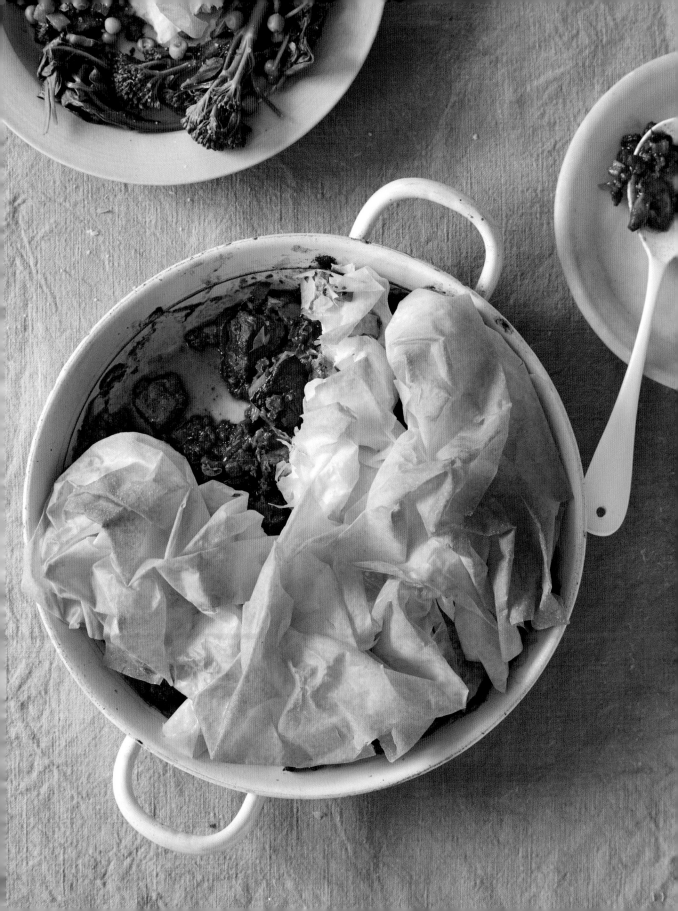

MEATY MUSHROOM PIE

This Joe Wicks-inspired pie is topped with phyllo pastry. It's hearty and filling, but is lower in fat, processed carbs, and calories (and cooks more quickly). Make sure your vegan meat is low in salt and saturated fat.

SERVES 4

1 onion
1 carrot
2 celery stalks
14 oz mixed mushrooms
10 sprigs fresh thyme
1 sprig fresh rosemary
10 sprigs fresh parsley
14 oz vegan meat
1½ tbsp olive oil
1 bay leaf
1 tbsp tomato paste
3 tbsp red wine
1 cup vegetable stock
4 sheets phyllo pastry
cooking oil spray

TO SERVE

7 oz broccolini
1½ cups frozen peas
7 oz fresh spinach leaves
1 lemon
salt and black pepper

PREHEAT OVEN TO 375°F | LARGE SKILLET | 7 X 11-INCH BAKING DISH | SAUCEPAN | BOILING WATER

First, prep the ingredients | Peel and dice the onion | Peel and dice the carrot | Trim and thinly slice the celery | Roughly chop the mushrooms | Pick the leaves from the thyme and rosemary sprigs, then roughly chop | Pick and roughly chop the parsley leaves | Cut the vegan meat into bite-sized chunks

Now, brown the vegan meat | Warm ½ tablespoon of the olive oil in the large skillet over medium heat | Add half the vegan meat and cook, stirring, for 3–4 minutes, until the chunks are browning | Transfer the browned chunks to a plate | Repeat this process with another ½ tablespoon of the olive oil and the remaining vegan meat

Make the pie filling | Heat the remaining ½ tablespoon of olive oil in the skillet over medium heat | Add the onion and a pinch of salt and cook, stirring, for 3–4 minutes | Add the carrot and celery and stir for 2 minutes | Add the mushrooms and stir for 3–4 minutes | Add the thyme, rosemary, and bay leaf and stir for 1 minute, until aromatic | Add the tomato paste and stir for another minute | Add the browned vegan meat and stir for 1 minute | Add the wine and stir for 1 minute | Add the stock, increase the heat, and simmer for about 10 minutes, until most of the liquid has evaporated | Add the parsley leaves | Taste and season to perfection with salt and pepper | Tip into the baking dish, smooth it out with the back of a spoon, and leave to cool for 5 minutes

Now, make the topping | Crumple the phyllo pastry sheets into loose balls and cover the top of the dish | Spray with 4 sprays of cooking spray | Bake in the oven for 20 minutes, until the pastry is crispy and beginning to darken

Five minutes before the pie is set to come out of the oven, trim the broccolini | Put the broccolini and peas in a saucepan, cover with boiling water, and allow to warm through for 3–4 minutes | Put the spinach in a colander, pour the broccolini and peas and all the hot water from the pan into the colander (this will wilt the spinach) | Halve the lemon | Squeeze a little lemon juice over the greens and season with salt and pepper | Portion the pie onto plates and serve immediately with the greens

521 KCAL | LOW FAT | LOW SUGAR | FULL OF FIBER | PROTEIN PACKED

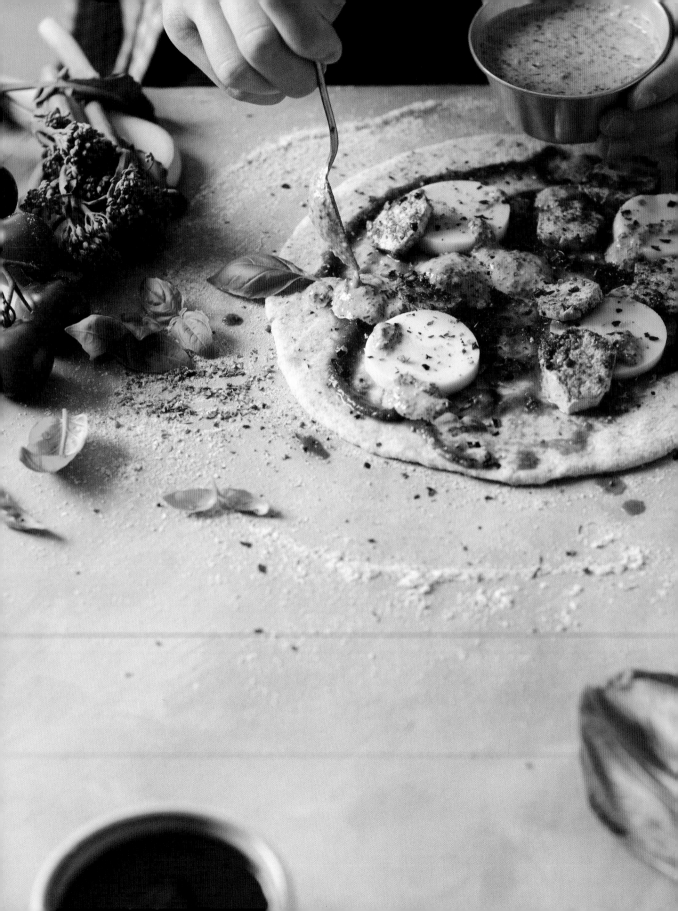

HEALTHIER PIZZA DOUGH

For many people, pizza is more than just a food—it's a way of life! And it's become something of an obsession for BOSH!, too. We've loved creating indulgent pizzas for our fans and our channel, so it was important for us that we could create a Healthy Vegan version. This pizza dough is much healthier than the kind you'll find in restaurants and stores, because we use a 50/50 dough. The white flour gives you the texture and flavor of a classic pizza crust, but the whole wheat flour makes it higher in fiber with a lower GI value.

MAKES ENOUGH DOUGH FOR 2 LARGE PIZZA CRUSTS (TO SERVE 4)

2 cups white
  bread flour, plus
  extra for dusting
2 cups whole wheat flour
1 tsp fine salt
1⅓ cups lukewarm water
1⅛ tsp (½ a 7g envelope)
  fast-action dried yeast
1 tbsp superfine sugar
vegetable oil or olive oil,
  for greasing

CLEAN WORK SURFACE DUSTED LIBERALLY WITH FLOUR | PLASTIC WRAP

Combine the flours and salt in a bowl | Make a well in the center of the mixture

Put the lukewarm water, yeast, and sugar in a measuring cup, mix well and leave to stand for about 5 minutes, until it's frothing, then pour into the well in the dry flour mixture | Stir with a fork, in a circular movement, to bring the flour in from the inner edge of the well and mix it into the water | Continue to mix, bringing in all the flour until the dough comes together | If there are still parts of the flour not combining, add a little splash of water to help the dough come together

Tip the dough out on the clean, flour-dusted surface | Knead it by rolling it backward and forward, using your hands to stretch, pull, and push the dough | Keep kneading for 10 minutes until you have a springy dough

Lightly grease a bowl with oil | Place the dough in the bowl, cover with oiled plastic wrap, and leave in a warm place to rise for about 1 hour, or until doubled in size | This is the first prove and your dough is now ready to make into one of the following recipes

PEPPERONI & PESTO PIZZA

It's always so much better to make your own pizzas—you can get them to taste exactly like you want and you'll be sure you're not getting any added unhealthy nonsense. We discovered that adding a few spices to smoked tofu results in an amazing plant-based pepperoni! Try it here with a super quick and delicious pesto topping. See photos on pages 164 and 170.

MAKES 2 PIZZAS (SERVES 4)

Healthier Pizza Dough (page 165)

all-purpose flour, for dusting

semolina, for dusting

⅔ cup canned tomato purée

1¾ oz vegan cheese (the meltier the better)

chile flakes, to taste

FOR THE TOFU "PEPPERONI"

10 oz firm smoked tofu

¼ tsp freshly ground black pepper

½ tsp garlic powder

½ tsp ground fennel seeds

½ tsp ground mustard seeds or mustard powder

¼ tsp cayenne pepper

½ tsp smoked paprika

2 tsp red wine (more to loosen, if needed)

1 tsp olive oil

FOR THE PESTO

1½ oz fresh basil sprigs, plus extra leaves to serve

1 small garlic clove

½ lemon

3 tbsp nutritional yeast

1 tbsp water

3 tbsp almonds

TOFU PRESS OR 2 CLEAN TEA TOWELS AND A WEIGHT SUCH AS A HEAVY BOOK | CLEAN WORK SURFACE DUSTED LIBERALLY WITH FLOUR | PLASTIC WRAP | PIZZA STONE OR HEAVY, LARGE BAKING SHEET | FOOD PROCESSOR OR BLENDER | ROLLING PIN | LARGE BAKING SHEET DUSTED WITH SEMOLINA

First, prep the tofu "pepperoni" | Press the tofu using a tofu press or place it between two clean tea towels, lay it on a plate, and put a weight on top | Leave for 15–20 minutes to drain off any liquid and firm up

Meanwhile, tip the risen dough onto the floured work surface | Knead for 1 minute to knock it back, then divide into two equal pieces | Flour each dough ball, cover with oiled plastic wrap, and leave to rest for 12–15 minutes (this will make the dough easier to roll)

Preheat the oven to 475°F | Put the pizza stone or heavy, large baking sheet on the middle rack of the oven to heat up | Dust the work surface with more flour

Cut the block of tofu in half lengthwise | Trim the corners of both halves of the tofu to make two roundish cylinders that are roughly the diameter of a quarter | Slice the cylinders into rounds a scant ¼ inch thick

Prepare the rub and season the tofu | Combine all the remaining "pepperoni" ingredients in a medium bowl and stir to combine, adding a little more red wine to loosen if needed | Add the tofu discs to the bowl and stir gently to ensure the paste is evenly coating the tofu | Set the bowl to one side and carry on with other prep

Make the pesto | Pick the basil leaves and discard the stems | Peel the garlic | Juice the half lemon | Put all the pesto ingredients in the food processor or blender, season with salt and pepper, and blitz | Loosen with a splash of water if necessary | Taste and season to perfection with salt and pepper

640 KCAL | LOW SUGAR | FULL OF FIBER | PROTEIN PACKED

1½ tbsp extra-virgin
   olive oil
salt and black pepper

TO SERVE
**chile flakes, optional
basil leaves, optional**

Now, build the pizzas | Roll one dough half out to make a pizza crust no more than a scant ¼ inch thick | Carefully roll it back onto the rolling pin and transfer to the baking sheet dusted with semolina | Ladle a liberal amount of tomato purée onto the pizza crust and swirl it around the dough evenly, almost up to the edge, with the bottom of the ladle | Decorate the pizza with half the "pepperoni" and grate over half the vegan cheese | Drizzle over generous helpings of the pesto

Cook the pizzas and serve! | Slide the baking sheet with the topped pizza crust onto the hot pizza stone or baking sheet in the oven and bake for 8–12 minutes, until the crust has started to lightly brown | Prepare the second pizza | Take the first pizza out of the oven, sprinkle with chile flakes, garnish with fresh basil, cut into slices, and serve | Repeat the process with the second pizza

TEXAS BBQ PIZZA

Who would have thought you could have a healthy Texas BBQ pizza? This has all the flavor of the indulgent original, but none of the bad bits. We use mushrooms for shredded chicken and smoked tofu for that bacon flavor. See photo on page 171.

MAKES 2 PIZZAS (SERVES 4)

Healthier Pizza Dough (page 165)

all-purpose flour, for dusting

semolina, for dusting

FOR THE TOPPING

5 oz firm smoked tofu

7 oz shiitake mushrooms

1 green bell pepper

3 scallions

12 cherry tomatoes

½ cup canned corn

4 tbsp BBQ sauce (low-sugar store-bought or use our BBQ Bourbon Sauce opposite)

chile flakes, to taste

FOR THE TOFU & MUSHROOM RUB

½ tbsp olive oil

½ tbsp smoked paprika

¼ tsp garlic powder

¼ tsp onion powder

pinch of cayenne pepper

¼ tsp dried oregano

1 tbsp BBQ sauce (low-sugar store-bought or use our BBQ Bourbon Sauce opposite)

pinch each of salt and black pepper

TOFU PRESS OR 2 CLEAN TEA TOWELS AND A WEIGHT SUCH AS A HEAVY BOOK | CLEAN WORK SURFACE DUSTED LIBERALLY WITH FLOUR | PLASTIC WRAP | PIZZA STONE OR HEAVY, LARGE BAKING SHEET | ROLLING PIN | LARGE BAKING SHEET DUSTED WITH SEMOLINA

First, press the tofu using a tofu press or place it between two clean tea towels, lay it on a plate, and put a weight on top | Leave for 15–20 minutes to drain off any liquid and firm up

Meanwhile, tip the risen dough onto the floured work surface | Knead for 1 minute to knock it back, then divide into two equal pieces | Flour each dough ball, cover with oiled plastic wrap, and leave to rest for 12–15 minutes (this will make the dough easier to roll)

Preheat the oven to 475°F | Put the pizza stone or heavy, large baking sheet on the middle rack of the oven | Dust the work surface with flour

Now, make the rub and flavor the toppings | Put all the rub ingredients in a bowl and stir to combine | Cut the pressed tofu into scant ¼-inch cubes and add to the bowl | Cut the shiitake mushrooms into thin matchsticks, add to the bowl, and toss well to combine

Prep the rest of the ingredients | Trim, halve, and core the green bell pepper, then cut it into ¼-inch-thick slices | Trim and thinly slice the scallions | Halve the cherry tomatoes | Rinse the corn, then dry it on paper towels

Now, build the pizzas | Roll one dough half out to make a pizza crust no more than a scant ¼ inch thick | Carefully roll it back onto the rolling pin and transfer to the baking sheet dusted with semolina | Liberally spread with BBQ sauce, leaving a 1-inch border around the edge | Top generously with smoked tofu, shiitake mushrooms, green pepper slices, cherry tomatoes, and corn | Sprinkle with scallions and chile flakes

Cook the pizzas! | Slide the baking sheet with the topped pizza onto the hot pizza stone or baking sheet in the oven | Bake for 8–10 minutes, until the crust starts to lightly brown | Prepare the second pizza | Take the first pizza out of the oven, slice, and serve | Cook the second pizza

591 KCAL | LOW FAT | LOW SUGAR | FULL OF FIBER | PROTEIN PACKED

BBQ BOURBON SAUCE

BBQ sauce is available everywhere these days, so many people don't realize how easy it is to make your own. It's so much more rewarding, because you can adjust the flavors to your taste—plus it never fails to impress when you bring a bottle of homemade BBQ sauce to the table! This recipe is much lower in sugar than a store-bought version, too. A splash of bourbon is traditional, but you can leave it out if you prefer.

MAKES ⅔ CUP

1 cup apple juice

6 tbsp canned tomato purée

2 tbsp bourbon

2 tbsp balsamic vinegar

½ tsp sea salt

2 tsp chipotle paste

2 tsp yellow mustard

2½ tbsp maple syrup

2 tsp yeast extract (e.g., Marmite)

1 tsp liquid smoke, optional

¼ tsp hot sauce (e.g., Tabasco), optional

salt and black pepper

MEDIUM SAUCEPAN | AIRTIGHT CONTAINER

Put all the ingredients, except the salt and pepper, in the saucepan | Put the saucepan over medium heat, whisk to combine, and simmer for 12–15 minutes, stirring occasionally to prevent the sauce catching | Add a little water to thin it out if it gets too thick | Season to taste with salt and pepper, remove the pan from the heat, and leave the sauce to cool to room temperature | Transfer the sauce to the airtight container, store in the fridge, and consume within 2 weeks

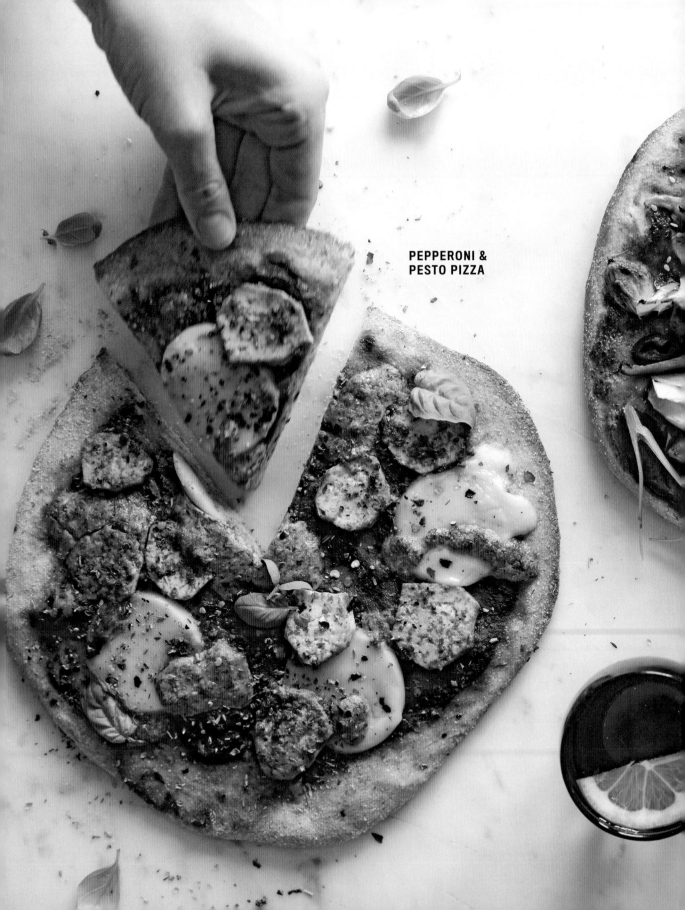

PEPPERONI &
PESTO PIZZA

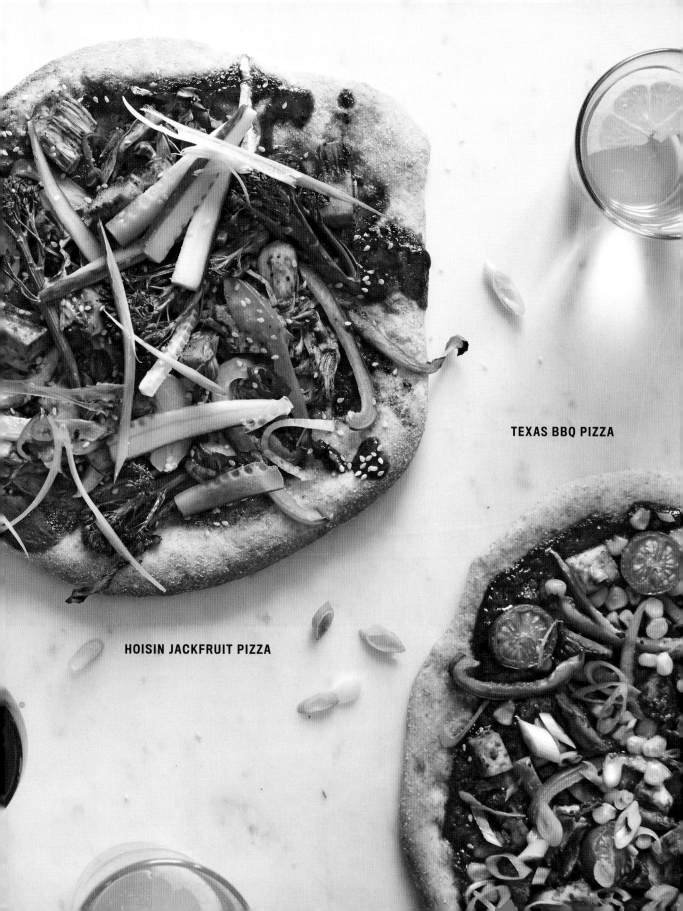

TEXAS BBQ PIZZA

HOISIN JACKFRUIT PIZZA

HOISIN JACKFRUIT PIZZA

For this pizza, we took flavor inspiration from classic Chinese duck pancakes, combining jackfruit with fresh scallions and cucumber. The hoisin sauce is the hero here though, with its sweet smoky umaminess. See photo on page 171.

MAKES 2 PIZZAS (SERVES 4)

Healthier Pizza Dough (page 165)

all-purpose flour, for dusting

semolina, for dusting

FOR THE TOPPING

generous ⅓ cup hoisin sauce (use store-bought or make our healthy Hoisin Sauce opposite)

1 (14 oz) can young green jackfruit in water

1 red bell pepper

1 fresh red chile

5 oz broccolini

1 head bok choy

2 scallions

¼ cucumber

2 tsp white sesame seeds

PREHEAT OVEN TO 475°F | CLEAN WORK SURFACE DUSTED LIBERALLY WITH FLOUR | PLASTIC WRAP | PIZZA STONE OR HEAVY, LARGE BAKING SHEET HEATING UP IN THE OVEN | LARGE BAKING SHEET DUSTED WITH SEMOLINA | ROLLING PIN

First, tip the risen dough onto the floured work surface | Knead for 1 minute to knock it back, then divide into two equal pieces | Flour each dough ball, cover with oiled plastic wrap, and leave to rest for 12–15 minutes (this will make the dough easier to roll)

Make your hoisin sauce (if using our recipe)

Now, prep the jackfruit | Drain the jackfruit, rinse under a cold tap, and pat dry with a clean tea towel or paper towels | Put the jackfruit in a bowl and shred the chunks with two forks | Add half the hoisin sauce to the bowl and fold to coat | Leave the jackfruit to marinate

While the jackfruit is marinating, prep the remaining toppings | Trim, halve, core, and thinly slice the red bell pepper | Rip the stem off the chile (remove seeds if you like) and thinly slice | Trim and halve the broccolini lengthwise to make long, thin strips | Trim and roughly chop the bok choy | Trim, halve and cut the scallions into ribbons | Cut the cucumber into fine matchsticks, discarding the watery seeds

Now, build the pizzas | Roll one dough half out to make a pizza crust no more than a scant ¼ inch thick | Carefully roll it back onto the rolling pin and transfer to the baking sheet dusted with semolina | Spread half the remaining hoisin sauce over the pizza crust in a thin layer with a large spoon, leaving a 1-inch border rim around the edge | Top the pizza with half the marinated jackfruit, chile, bell pepper, broccolini, and bok choy

Cook the pizzas and serve! | Slide the baking sheet with the topped pizza base onto the hot pizza stone or baking sheet in the oven and bake for 8–10 minutes until the crust has started to lightly brown | Prepare the second pizza | Take the first pizza out of the oven and scatter with half the scallions, cucumber, and sesame seeds | Cut into slices and serve | Repeat the process with the second pizza

628 KCAL | LOW FAT | LOW SUGAR | FULL OF FIBER | PROTEIN PACKED

HOISIN SAUCE

"Hoisin" actually comes from the Cantonese word for seafood, but it's now synonymous with a specific flavor of Chinese cooking. This delicious sauce re-creates it perfectly, and would go well with Mandarin pancakes, in a stir-fry, or as a dip for spring rolls.

MAKES GENEROUS ⅓ CUP

2½ tbsp superfine sugar

2 tbsp water

1 tbsp Chinese black bean sauce

1 tbsp soy sauce

1 tbsp rice vinegar

4 prunes

½ tsp sesame oil

½ tsp Chinese five-spice

1 tsp sriracha

BLENDER | AIRTIGHT CONTAINER

Put all the ingredients in the blender and blitz until smooth | Taste and tweak to perfection | Store in the fridge in an airtight container | The sauce will keep for up to 1 week

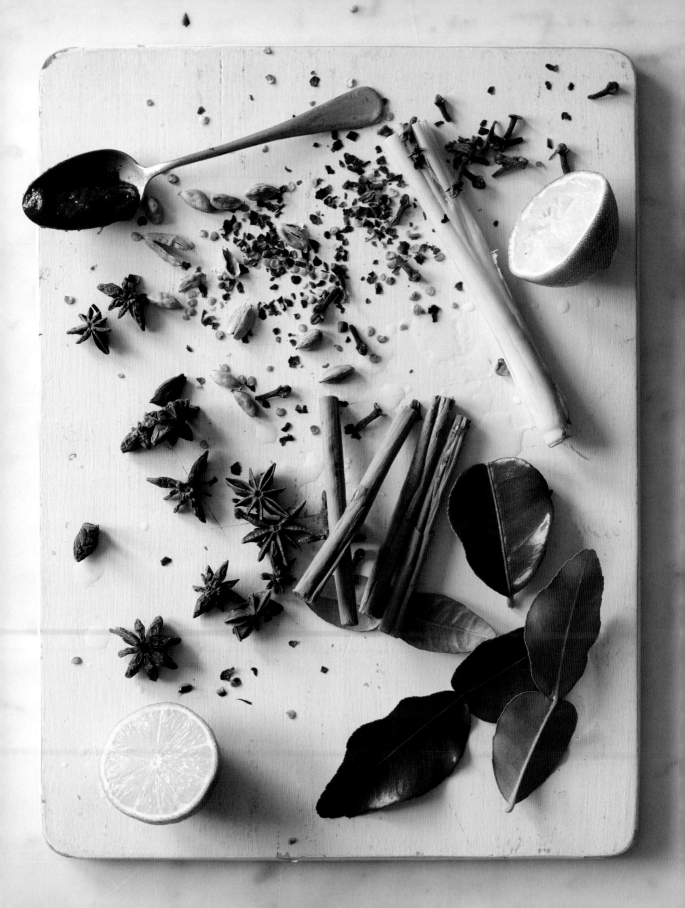

LEGENDARY RENDANG

With the help of our buddy Liam Chau, we created a healthier version of this true Asian classic. Using drinking coconut milk reduces the saturated fat content, and the eggplant is melt-in-the-mouth and coated in a wonderfully luxurious and thick gravy. The flavors that run through this rendang are full, robust, and traditional.

SERVES 2

1 large eggplant
½ tbsp vegetable oil
3 green cardamom pods
1 unwaxed lime
2 tsp tamarind paste
3 dried kaffir lime leaves
1 tbsp maple syrup
1 tsp dark soy sauce
2 tbsp unsweetened shredded coconut
salt

FOR THE COCONUT BÉCHAMEL

1¼ cups store-bought coconut milk beverage
3 whole cloves
3 star anise
1 cinnamon stick
1 lemongrass stalk
½ tbsp vegetable oil
1 tbsp all-purpose flour

FOR THE RENDANG PASTE

5 oz shallots
3 garlic cloves
¾ oz fresh ginger
2 lemongrass stalks
1 tsp chile flakes
1 tsp tamarind paste
3 tbsp water

ingredients list and recipe continued . . .

PREHEAT OVEN TO 400°F | 3 MEDIUM SAUCEPANS | LINE A SHEET PAN WITH PARCHMENT PAPER | BLENDER

First, infuse the coconut beverage for the béchamel | Heat the coconut beverage in one of the medium saucepans over medium heat until warm, then remove from the heat and add the cloves, star anise, cinnamon stick, and lemongrass stalk | Leave to infuse for 3–4 minutes

Now, prep the eggplant | Trim the eggplant and quarter it lengthwise, then cut each quarter into 1-inch chunks | Spread the eggplant chunks out on the lined sheet pan, drizzle over a little of the vegetable oil, season with a little salt, and toss to coat | Put the pan in the oven and roast for 15–20 minutes, until cooked

Now, make the béchamel | Remove the cloves, star anise, cinnamon stick, and lemongrass from the infused coconut drink | Heat the vegetable oil in the second saucepan over medium heat | Add the flour and stir it into the oil (it will clump slightly–don't worry) | Gradually add the coconut beverage, whisking constantly, until the sauce is smooth and thick | Remove from the heat and set to one side

Make the rendang paste | Peel and halve the shallots | Peel the garlic | Peel the ginger by scraping off the skin with a spoon | Peel away the hard outer bark of the lemongrass stalks | Trim the stalks and bash with a pestle to release the oils | Put the shallots, garlic, ginger, lemongrass, chile flakes, tamarind paste, and water in the blender and blitz to form a smooth and lightly textured paste

Now, prep the rest of the ingredients | Crush the cardamom pods and remove the papery husks | Zest and halve the lime

597 KCAL | LOW FAT | LOW SUGAR | FULL OF FIBER

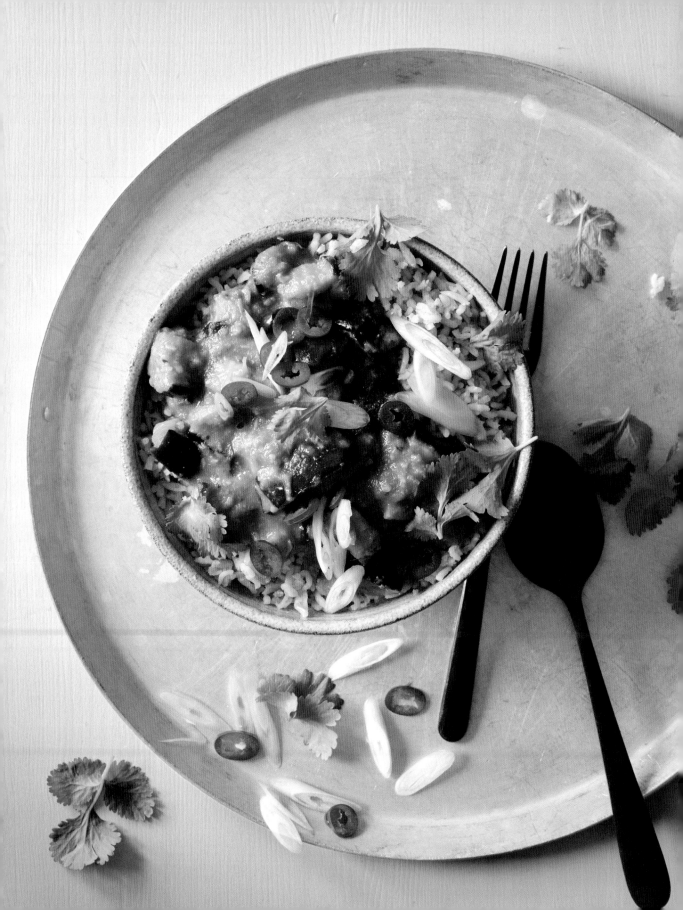

. . . continued from previous page

TO SERVE

1 scallion

1 fresh red chilli

4 cups cooked basmati rice or 2 (8.8 oz) bags microwavable brown basmati rice

small handful of cilantro leaves, optional

Now, make the rendang | Heat the remaining vegetable oil in the third saucepan over medium heat, add the cardamom seeds, and stir until aromatic | Add the rendang paste and stir for 3–4 minutes until very aromatic | Add the roasted eggplant pieces and stir to coat them in the paste | Add the béchamel, tamarind paste, lime leaves, maple syrup, and soy sauce and cook, stirring, for 4–5 minutes, loosening the sauce with up to 3 tablespoons of water if necessary | Add the shredded coconut and fold it into the sauce | Add the lime zest and half the juice | Taste the rendang and season to perfection with salt

Prepare to serve | Trim and thinly slice the scallions | Rip the stem from the chile, seed, and thinly slice | Heat the rice, if necessary, or cook it following the package instructions | Plate up the rice, top with the rendang, garnish with scallions, chile, cilantro, and extra lime juice, to taste

NOT-THAT-NAUGHTY BURGER
WITH FRISBEE FRIES

This healthy burger is so good we've put it on the cover! Along with our own tasty vegan burger, we've created a healthier but still delicious burger sauce and a smoky relish that's sweet but contains no added sugar. Serve with Frisbee fries and, well, you know what? Burgers have never tasted so good.

MAKES 2

FOR THE SMOKY RELISH

½ small red onion
1 small garlic clove
1 small fresh red chile
5 oz cherry tomatoes
½ tbsp olive oil
¼ tsp smoked paprika
½ tbsp tomato paste
1 tsp soy sauce
¼ tsp maple syrup
½ lime
salt and black pepper

FOR THE BURGER PATTIES

4½ oz sweet potato
½ onion
2 tbsp olive oil
scant ½ cup cooked
   brown rice
1 tbsp breadcrumbs
pinch of salt
pinch of ground
   black pepper
pinch of ground cumin
pinch of garlic powder
pinch of smoked paprika
2 tsp all-purpose flour
¾ cup canned black
   beans

ingredients list and recipe
continued . . .

PREHEAT OVEN TO 400°F | LINE 2 SHEET PANS WITH PARCHMENT PAPER | FINE GRATER OR MICROPLANE | MEDIUM SKILLET | FOOD PROCESSOR

First, make the smoky relish | Peel and dice the red onion | Peel and grate the garlic | Rip the stem from the chile, halve it lengthwise, remove the seeds, then finely dice | Quarter the tomatoes

Heat the olive oil in the skillet over medium heat | Add the onion and a pinch of salt and cook, stirring, for 4–5 minutes | Add the garlic and chile and stir for 1 minute | Add the tomatoes, smoked paprika, tomato paste, and soy sauce | Stir the ingredients together and simmer for 15 minutes, stirring occasionally to prevent the relish catching at the bottom of the pan | Add the maple syrup | Remove from the heat, squeeze the lime juice into the relish, taste, and season to perfection with salt and pepper | Transfer to a bowl and set aside, and wipe out the pan

Next, cook the sweet potato for the burger patties | Peel the sweet potato and cut into ¾-inch cubes, put on one of the lined sheet pans and bake for 30 minutes

Now, make the Frisbee fries | Slice the new potatoes into discs ⅛ inch thick | Add the olive oil to a mixing bowl along with a pinch of salt and pepper and some chile flakes | Put the potato slices in the bowl and toss to coat | Spread the potato slices out on the other lined sheet pan, put the pan in the oven, and bake with the sweet potato for 20–25 minutes, turning them once after 15 minutes, until golden and crispy

Meanwhile, make the burger sauce | Put all the ingredients in a bowl and stir to combine | Put the sauce to one side

682 KCAL | LOW FAT | LOW SUGAR | FULL OF FIBER | PROTEIN PACKED

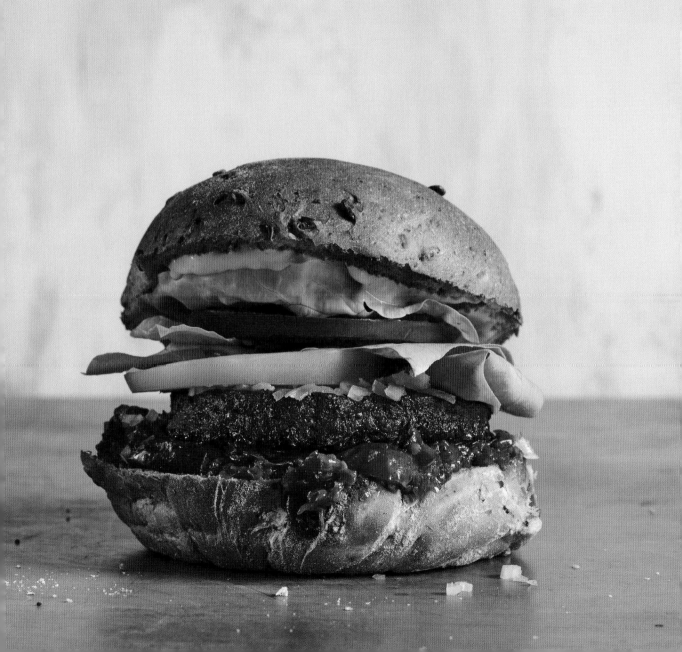

. . . continued from previous page

FOR THE FRISBEE FRIES

5 oz new potatoes

½ tbsp olive oil

chile flakes, to taste

FOR THE BURGER SAUCE

1½ tbsp plant-based yogurt

½ tsp sriracha

¼ tsp yellow mustard

½ tsp red wine vinegar

TO SERVE

¾ oz dairy-free cheese

1 beefsteak tomato (or slices from 2 different color beefsteak tomatoes)

1 small shallot

2 medium whole wheat burger buns (about 3 oz each)

4 lettuce leaves

Peel and finely chop the onion for the burger mixture | Pour half the oil into the clean skillet | Add the onion and fry for 8–10 minutes, until very soft | Transfer the onion to a large bowl and wipe out the pan

Remove the sweet potato and fries from the oven and keep the fries warm

Now, make the burger patties | Put the baked sweet potato in the food processor | Add the rice, breadcrumbs, salt, pepper, cumin, garlic powder, smoked paprika, and flour | Rinse the black beans, add them to the food processor, then whizz to a thick paste | Scrape the paste into the bowl with the onion and mix everything together with a spoon | Add the remaining oil to the pan and put it over medium-high heat | Divide the burger mixture into two and use your hands to mold them into patty shapes | Place the patties in the hot pan and fry for 3 minutes on each side, until golden

While the burgers are cooking, preheat the broiler | Grate the dairy-free cheese | Cut two ¼-inch-thick slices from the tomato(es), keeping the remaining tomato for another recipe | Peel and finely chop the shallot | Sprinkle the dairy-free cheese on the burgers in the pan during the last minute of cooking, so it melts | Cut the burger buns in half and toast under the broiler, cut side up, for 1 minute, until golden

Time to build the burgers and serve | Spread a teaspoon of burger sauce over the cut side of the top half of the burger bun | Spread 1½ tablespoons of relish on the bottom half (if you have any left over, put it in an airtight container in the fridge and eat within 5 days) | Place the burgers on the relish-covered bottom half of each bun | Sprinkle over the finely diced shallot | Lay the tomato slices and lettuce over the burgers | Close the lids of the burgers and plate them up | Take the fries out of the oven, plate them up with the burgers, and serve immediately

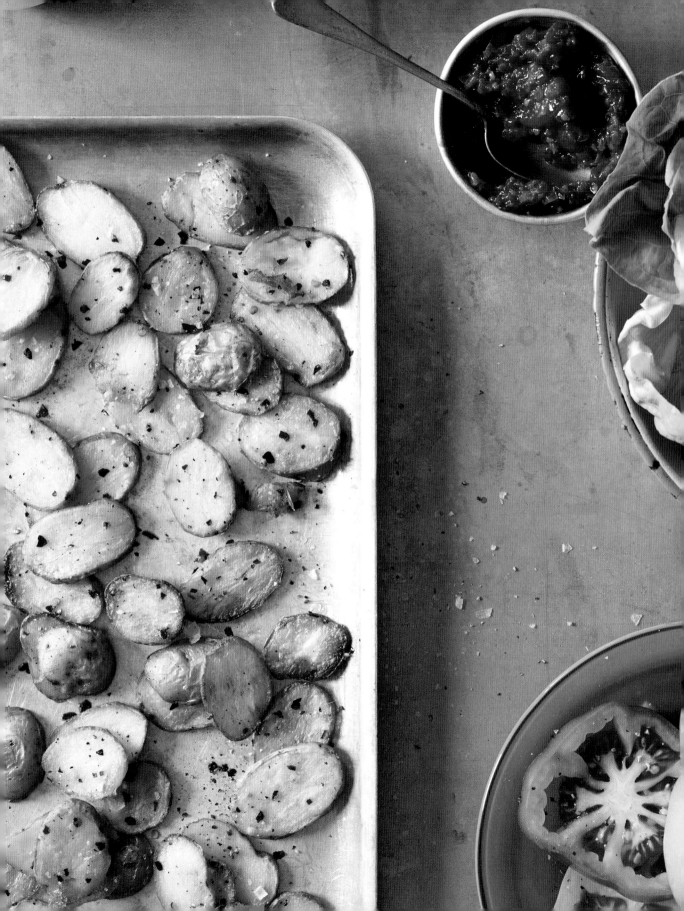

MEATBALLS WITH MASH & GRAVY

The flavor of these meatballs is just like traditional Italian meatballs, and the texture offers a really satisfying bite. You can even use the same technique to make some delicious sausages or burgers. Be aware that the wetness of the mixture will vary depending on the brand of burger patty you use; simply adjust with a little more flour if necessary.

SERVES 4

FOR THE MEATBALLS

8 sprigs fresh parsley

1 small garlic clove

1 (14 oz) can black beans

2 vegan burger patties (about 7 oz each), thawed if frozen

¼ tsp freshly ground black pepper

½ tsp dried oregano

¼ tsp chile flakes

1–1⅓ cups all-purpose flour

FOR THE GRAVY

1 red onion

1 carrot

1 celery stalk

2 garlic cloves

1 sprig fresh rosemary

2 sprigs fresh thyme

1 tbsp olive oil

1 tsp yeast extract (e.g., Marmite)

1½ tbsp balsamic vinegar

1 tbsp tomato paste

1 tbsp all-purpose flour

1⅔ cups vegetable stock

ingredients list and recipe continued . . .

PREHEAT OVEN TO 425°F | LINE A SHEET PAN WITH PARCHMENT PAPER | FOOD PROCESSOR | FINE GRATER OR MICROPLANE | SMALL SAUCEPAN | MEDIUM SAUCEPAN | STEAMER BASKET OR COLANDER | POTATO MASHER

First, make the meatballs | Pick and finely chop the parsley leaves | Peel the garlic | Drain and rinse the black beans, put them in the food processor with the burger patties, parsley, garlic, pepper, oregano, chile flakes, generous 1 cup of the flour, and a pinch of salt and pulse until all the ingredients are combined and a chunky paste is formed | If the mixture feels too wet to handle, add more flour | Roll the mixture into 20 equal-sized balls | Put the balls on the lined sheet pan, put the pan in the oven, and bake for 12–15 minutes, until cooked through | Turn off the oven but keep the balls in the oven to keep warm

Now, make the gravy | Peel and finely dice the red onion | Peel and coarsely grate the carrot | Trim and thinly slice the celery | Peel and grate the garlic | Pick the leaves from the rosemary and thyme sprigs and finely chop

Heat the olive oil in the small saucepan over medium heat | Add the onion and a pinch of salt to the pan and cook, stirring, for 3–4 minutes | Add the carrot and celery and stir for 3–4 minutes | Add the garlic, rosemary, and thyme and stir for another minute | Add the yeast extract, balsamic vinegar, and tomato paste and stir for 1 minute | Add the flour and stir for 1 minute | Add the vegetable stock to the pan, stir, bring to a boil, reduce the heat, and simmer for 20–30 minutes, until the gravy has thickened and reduced by about half

678 KCAL | LOW FAT | LOW SUGAR | FULL OF FIBER | PROTEIN PACKED

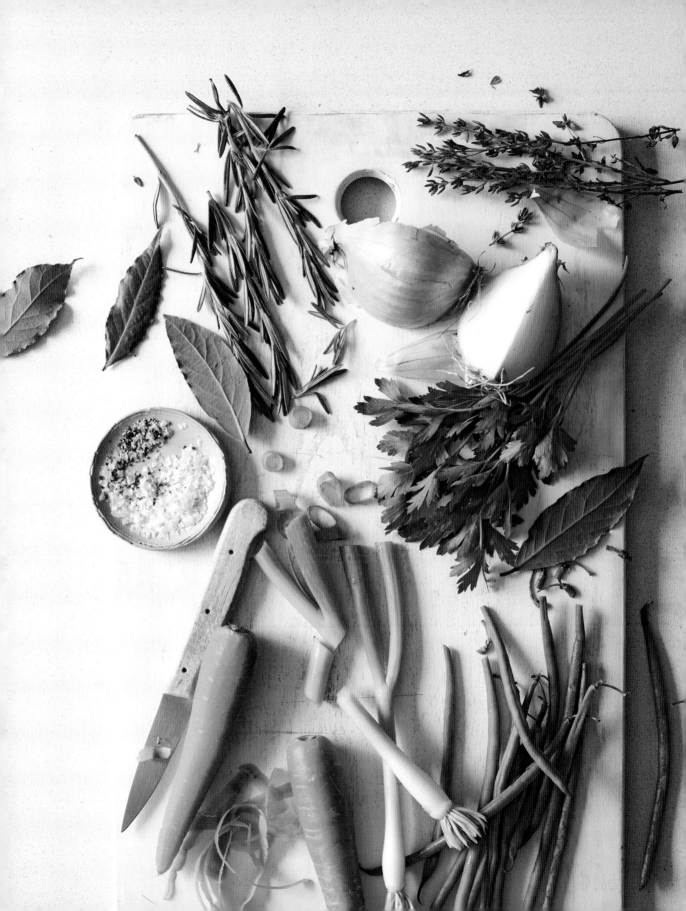

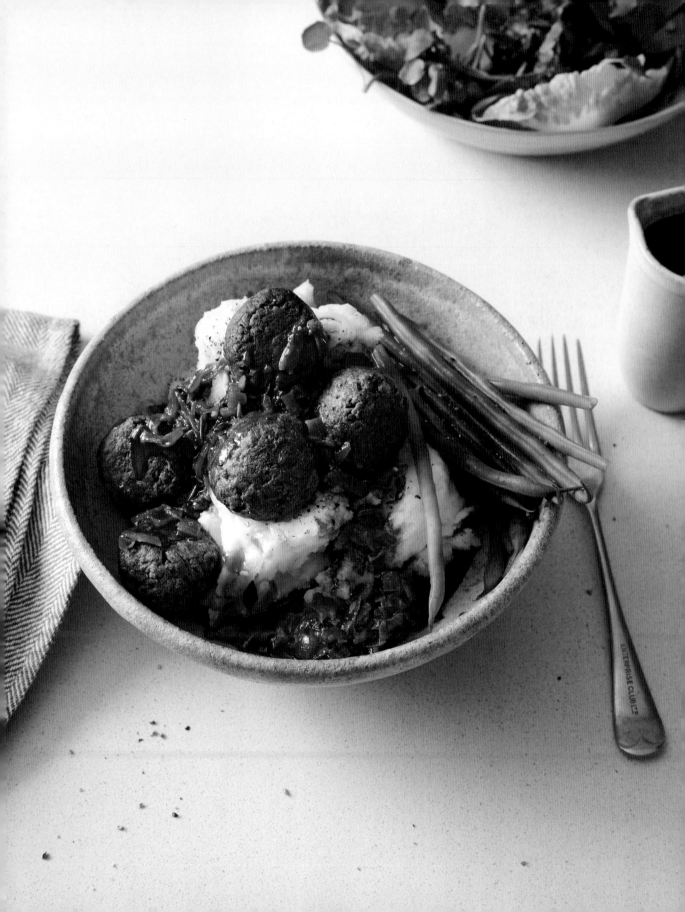

. . . continued from previous page

FOR THE MASH

3 scallions

4 russet potatoes (about 1 lb 10 oz)

5 tbsp oat milk

salt and black pepper

TO SERVE

4 oz green beans

3½ oz salad greens

While the gravy is simmering, boil the potatoes | Trim and thinly slice the scallions | Peel the potatoes and cut them into quarters | Put the potatoes and a pinch of salt in the medium saucepan and cover with cold water | Bring to a boil over high heat and cook the potatoes for 10 minutes, until tender

Quickly prep the green beans | Trim the green beans | Put the beans in the steamer basket or colander and place it over the saucepan of potatoes, put a lid on the basket or colander, and let the steam from the potatoes cook the beans for 2 minutes, until tender but still al dente | Remove the steamer from the pan

Now, finish the mash | Take the pan off the heat and drain the water from the potatoes | Use a potato masher to mash the potatoes, then stir in the oat milk | Taste and season to perfection with salt and pepper | Add the scallions to the pan, fold them in to combine and keep warm on the stove over low heat

Time to serve | Serve up the mash with the meatballs, green beans, and gravy | Season to taste with salt and pepper and serve immediately, with a handful of salad greens

CRISPY, STICKY TOFU
WITH BOK CHOY WOK-TOSSED RICE

This dish reminds us of all the best Chinese takeout we've ever eaten! The tofu is crispy and delicious yet still light and fluffy on the inside, and the sauce is rich, spicy, and sweet. You'll never need Chinese takeout again.

SERVES 2

FOR THE CRISPY TOFU

7 oz firm tofu
¼ cup cornstarch
cooking oil spray

FOR THE SAUCE

2-inch piece fresh ginger
2 large garlic cloves
1 fresh red chile
1 tbsp water
1 tsp cornstarch
1 tsp sesame oil
1 tbsp rice vinegar
2½ tbsp maple syrup
1 tbsp soy sauce

FOR THE BOK CHOY WOK-TOSSED RICE

1 (8.8 oz) bag microwaveable brown basmati rice
2 heads bok choy
1 garlic clove
1 tsp sesame oil
1 tsp soy sauce
pinch of chile flakes
1 scallion
1 tsp white sesame seeds

PREHEAT OVEN TO 425°F | LINE A SHEET PAN WITH PARCHMENT PAPER | TOFU PRESS OR 2 CLEAN TEA TOWELS AND A WEIGHT SUCH AS A HEAVY BOOK | FINE GRATER OR MICROPLANE | MEDIUM SKILLET | WOK

First, prep and roast the tofu | Press the tofu using a tofu press or place it between two clean tea towels, lay it on a plate, and put a weight on top | Leave for at least 30 minutes to drain off any liquid and firm up | Cut the tofu into ⅓-inch-thick batons | Roll the tofu in the cornstarch, until well coated | Spray the lined sheet pan with 4 sprays of cooking oil spray | Space out the coated tofu pieces on the pan | Spray the tops lightly with cooking spray | Bake in the oven for 15 minutes | Take the pan out, turn the pieces over, spray with a little more cooking spray, then bake for another 15 minutes

Meanwhile, prep the sauce | Peel the ginger by scraping off the skin with a spoon, then grate it | Peel and grate the garlic | Rip the stem from the chile, cut it in half lengthwise, and remove the seeds, then thinly slice | Mix the water and cornstarch in a glass to form a slurry | Warm the sesame oil in the medium skillet over medium heat | Add the garlic, ginger, and chile and cook for 1 minute, stirring | Add the rice vinegar, maple syrup and soy sauce and simmer gently, stirring, for 1 minute | Add the cornstarch slurry, stir it into the sauce, reduce the heat and simmer, stirring constantly, for 1 minute, until slightly thickened | Remove the pan from the heat

Cook and stir-fry the rice and bok choy | Cook the rice following the package instructions | Trim and slice the bok choy into very thin slivers | Peel and grate the garlic | Heat the oil in the wok over medium-high heat | Add the garlic and stir for 1 minute | Add the bok choy and toss for 2–3 minutes, until slightly softened | Stir in the cooked rice | Add the soy sauce and chile flakes and toss to combine

Finish and serve | Trim and thinly slice the scallions | Bring the sauce in the skillet up to a simmer | Add the crispy roast tofu and coat evenly | Plate up the rice, top with the crispy tofu, garnish with scallions and sesame seeds, and serve

622 KCAL | LOW SUGAR | FULL OF FIBER | PROTEIN PACKED

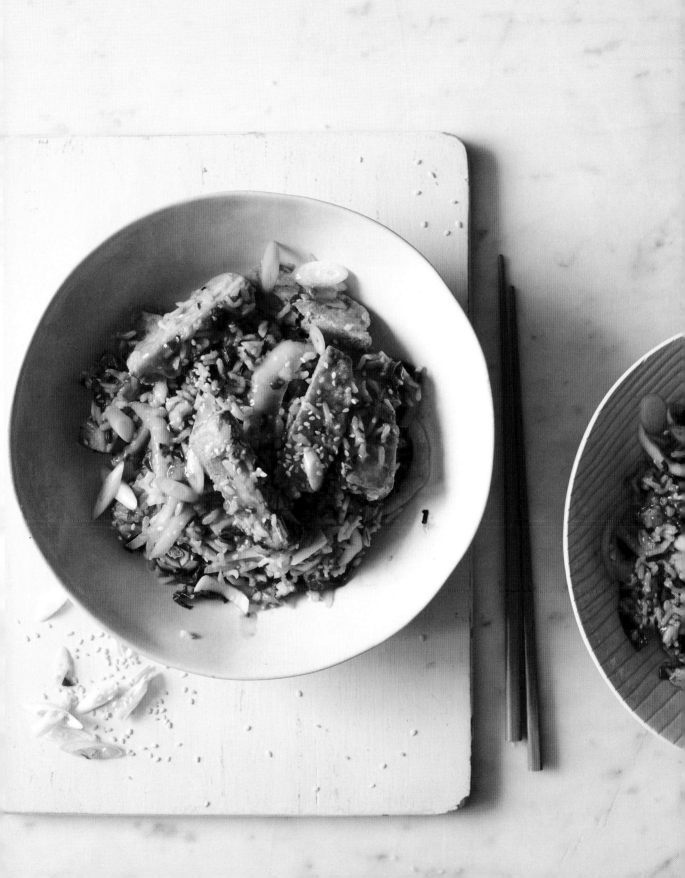

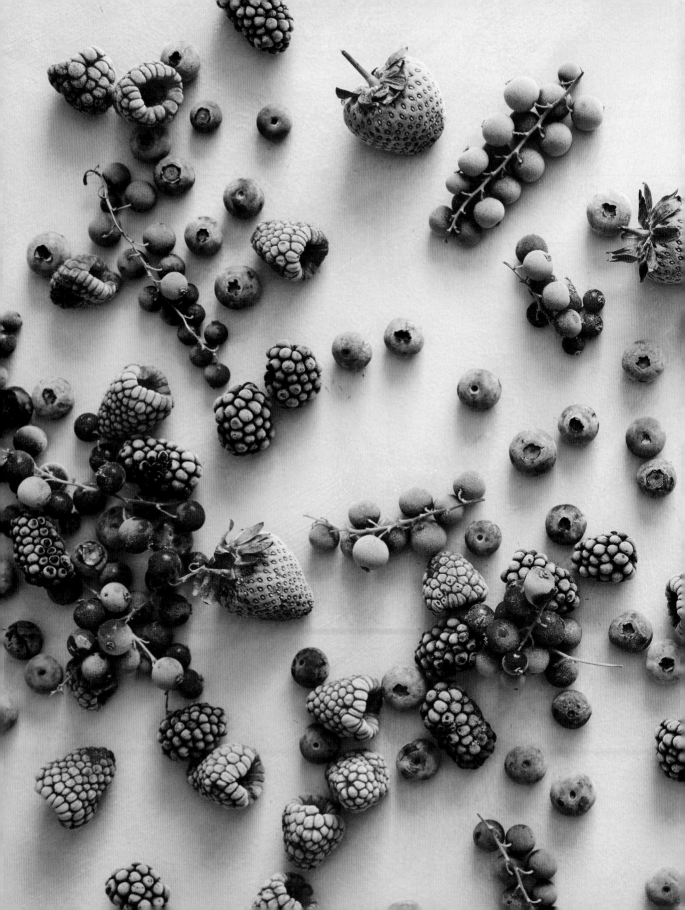

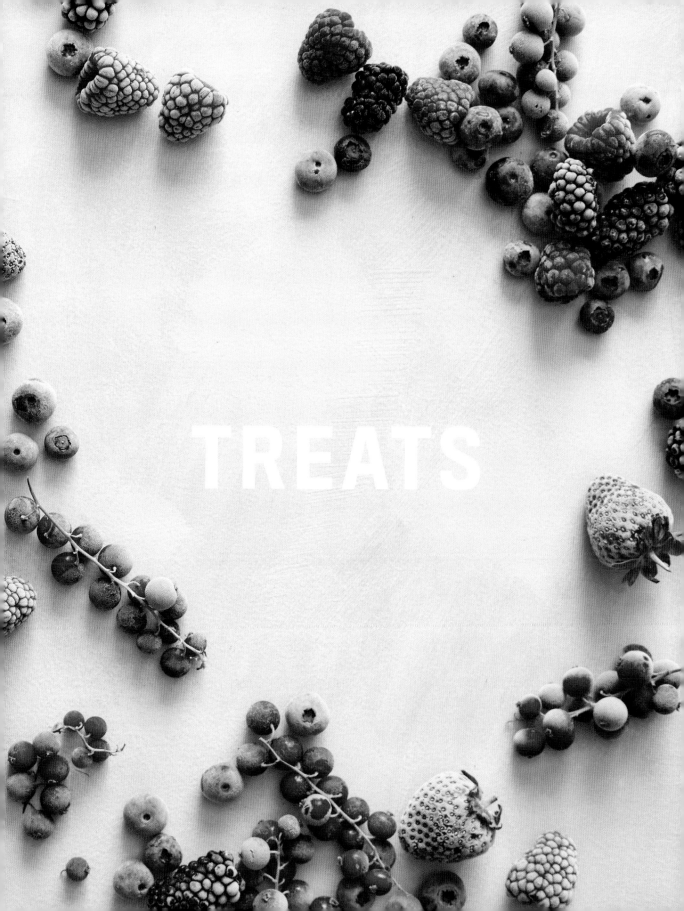

TREATS

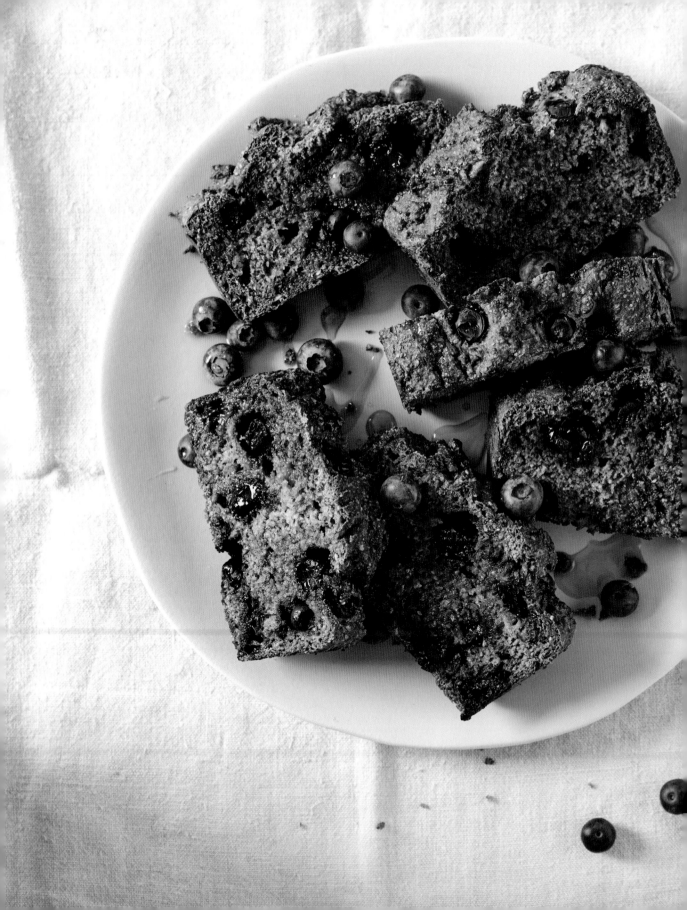

ANNA'S BLUEBERRY TOAST LOAF

Anna, our housemate, is an all-around culinary whiz and excels at delicious plant-based desserts. Sweet and moreish, and made with no added sugar, this high-fiber blueberry and banana loaf is the perfect breakfast (or even dessert!). We like to cut a big chunky slice and toast it, but it's also good cold.

SERVES 6

3 ripe bananas

½ cup unsweetened plant-based yogurt

1 tsp vanilla extract

1⅔ whole wheat flour

1 tsp baking soda

1 tsp baking powder

1 tsp ground cinnamon

pinch of salt

⅔ cup fresh blueberries, plus extra to serve, optional

maple syrup, to serve

PREHEAT OVEN TO 350°F | SPRAY A 2 LB LOAF PAN WITH COOKING SPRAY AND LINE IT WITH PARCHMENT PAPER

First, prep the wet and dry ingredients | Peel the bananas, put them in a mixing bowl, and mash until smooth | Add the yogurt and vanilla extract to the bowl and stir to mix | Put the flour, baking soda, baking powder, cinnamon, and salt in a separate bowl and stir to combine

Now, blend the mixtures together | Sift the dry mix into the wet mix and fold to combine | Add the blueberries and fold them into the batter | Pour the batter into the loaf pan and evenly spread the surface of the batter with a spatula

Put the pan in the oven | Bake the loaf for 50 minutes, or until a skewer inserted into the middle of the loaf comes out clean | Take the loaf out of the oven and let it cool to room temperature | Take the cake out of the pan and cut it into slices | Toast the slices before eating, drizzling them with a little maple syrup and extra blueberries if you like, and enjoy with a cup of tea

177 KCAL | LOW FAT | FULL OF FIBER | PROTEIN PACKED

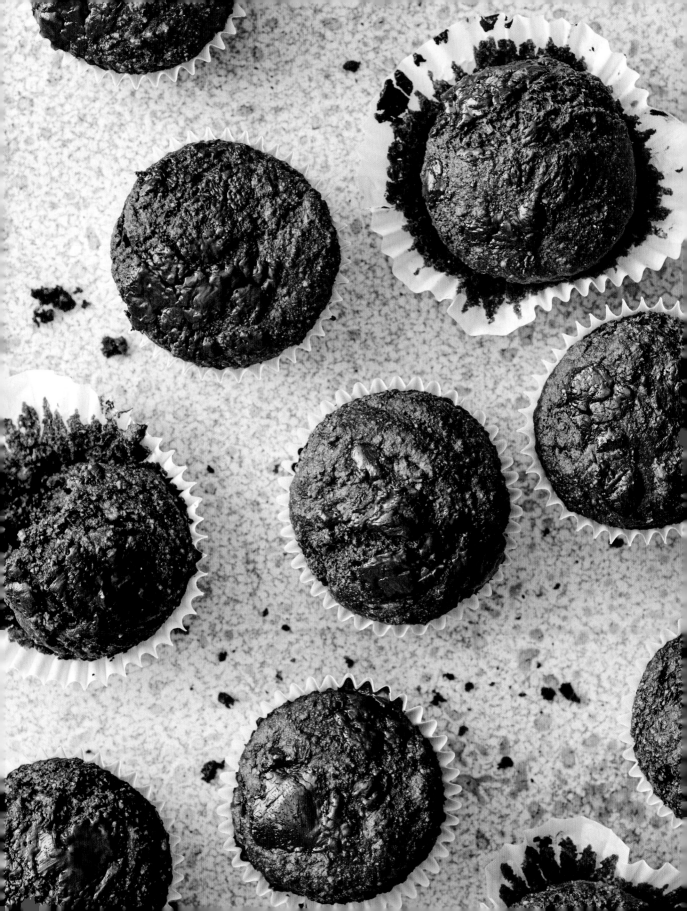

CHOCOLATE & BANANA MUFFINS

These decadent muffins combine the richness of dark chocolate with sweetness of banana, while a pinch of salt brings out those delicious contrasting flavors. Using whole wheat flour also makes them a healthier choice.

MAKES 12 MUFFINS

2½ oz dark chocolate

3 ripe bananas (about 12 oz unpeeled)

½ cup plus 1 tbsp unsweetened plant-based yogurt

6 tbsp maple syrup

7 tbsp unsweetened plant-based milk

2 tsp vanilla extract

2 cups whole wheat flour

3 tbsp unsweetened cocoa powder

1 tsp baking soda

1 tsp baking powder

½ tsp salt

½ tsp ground cinnamon

PREHEAT OVEN TO 350°F | 12-CUP MUFFIN PAN | 12 MUFFIN LINERS | COOLING RACK

First, prep the muffin batter | Chop the chocolate into chunks | Peel the bananas and mash them in a mixing bowl | Add the yogurt, maple syrup, milk, and vanilla extract to the bowl and mix together to combine | Sift the flour and combine it with the cocoa powder, baking soda, baking powder, salt, and cinnamon | Add the flour and cocoa mixture and chocolate chunks to the wet ingredients and fold together to form a batter

Now, bake the muffins | Line the cups of the muffin pan with the muffin liners | Transfer equal amounts of the muffin batter into each muffin cup | Put the pan in the oven and bake the muffins for 20–25 minutes, until the tops of muffins are puffed up and a skewer inserted into the middle of a muffin comes out clean | Leave to cool to room temperature then transfer the muffins to the cooling rack

174 KCAL | FULL OF FIBER

SALTED CARAMEL APPLE CRUMBLE & CUSTARD

We made everyone's favorite crumble healthy! Banana helps bind the topping together, instead of butter or other fats, and this also reduces the amount of added sugar needed. Plus this is the easiest vegan custard ever!

SERVES 6

PREHEAT OVEN TO 350°F | FOOD PROCESSOR | BOILING WATER | LARGE SAUCEPAN | 8-INCH SQUARE BAKING DISH | MEDIUM SAUCEPAN

FOR THE TOPPING

1 ripe banana
½ cup pecans
1 tsp ground cinnamon
1 tbsp canola oil
3 tbsp maple syrup
1¼ cups rolled oats
¾ cup whole wheat flour
pinch of salt

FOR THE FILLING

3½ oz Medjool dates
½ cup boiling water
½ tsp flaky salt
1 lb 12 oz apples
2 tbsp maple syrup
2 tbsp water
1 tsp ground cinnamon

FOR THE CUSTARD

2 tbsp cornstarch
1 tbsp water
2 cups plus 2 tbsp unsweetened plant-based milk
small pinch of ground turmeric
1 tbsp maple syrup
2 tsp vanilla extract

First, make the crumble topping | Peel the banana, put it in a bowl, and mash it really well with the back of a fork | Roughly chop the pecans | Add the cinnamon, oil, and maple syrup and stir to combine | Add the oats, flour, chopped pecans, and salt | Fold to combine, using your fingers to give a varied texture of large and small pieces

Now, prep the caramel | Pit the dates, put them in the food processor with the boiling water and salt, and pulse until you have a smooth caramel

Now, prep the apples | Core, peel, and thinly slice the apples | Put the apples in the large saucepan with the maple syrup and toss to coat | Add the water and cinnamon, place over medium heat and simmer for 8–10 minutes, stirring occasionally to help the apples soften evenly | Add the caramel to the pan and fold it into the apples

Build the crumble | Pour the apple filling into the baking dish, sprinkle over the crumble topping (you may have a couple of spoonfuls of crumble left over), put the dish in the oven, and bake for 25 minutes, until the crumble is crispy and golden

While the crumble is baking, make the custard | Put cornstarch and water in a small bowl and stir to form a slurry | Add half the milk and the turmeric to the bowl and stir to combine | Warm the remaining milk in the medium saucepan over medium heat, stirring continuously until it reaches a gentle simmer | Add the maple syrup and vanilla extract to the pan and stir to combine | Gently pour the cornstarch-milk mixture into the pan, whisking constantly, and cook for 5–7 minutes, until the custard is thick and smooth | Take the pan off the heat and pour the custard into a heatproof serving pitcher

Time to serve | Remove the crumble from the oven and serve immediately with the custard

429 KCAL | FULL OF FIBER

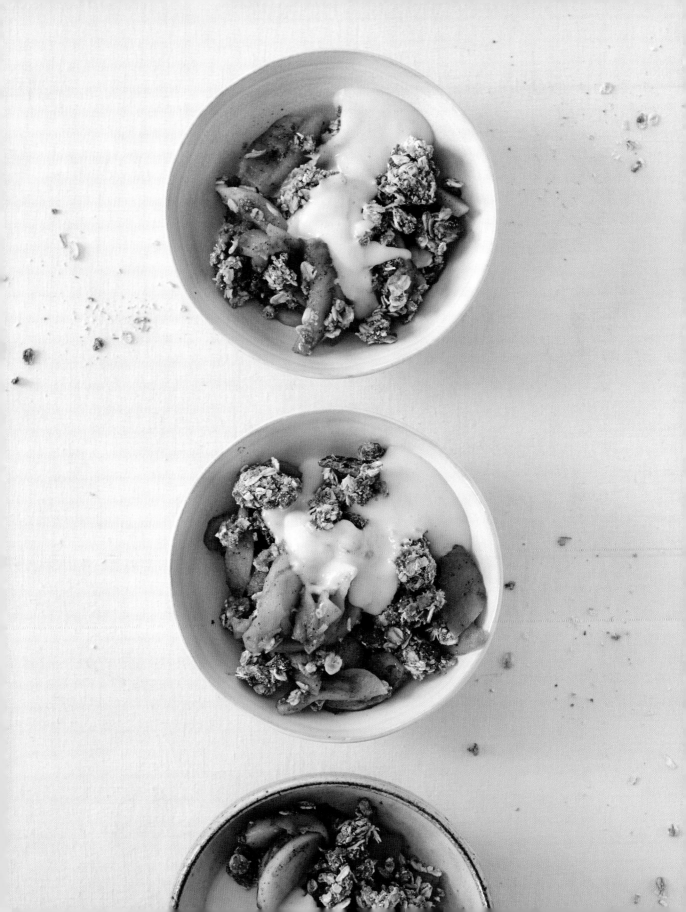

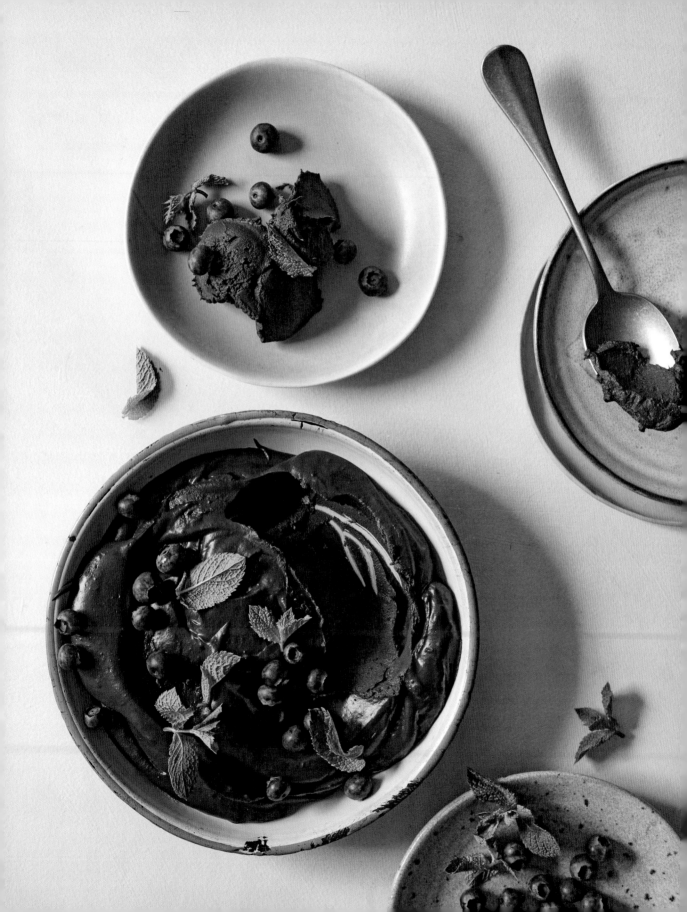

BANANA & CHOCOLATE MOUSSE

If you have any bananas in your fruit bowl that are overripe, this is the recipe for you. These mousse pots are rich and decadent and taste expensive. If you are hosting a dinner party and want to wow your buddies, give them a whirl! If you like it sweeter, add a little more maple syrup, but it will up the calories! It's important to allow time to chill the mousse before eating, so it has time to thicken.

SERVES 4

3 ripe bananas (10 oz peeled weight)
⅔ cup oat cream
¼ tsp ground cinnamon
5 tbsp maple syrup
1¾ cups unsweetened cocoa powder
⅓ cup fresh blueberries
handful of mint leaves

BLENDER

Prep the ingredients and blitz | Peel and roughly chop the bananas | Put the bananas, oat cream, cinnamon, and maple syrup in the blender and blitz until smooth | Add the cocoa powder and blitz again until smooth

Time to chill, garnish, and serve | Transfer the mousse to a dish or individual serving glasses and chill for at least 30 minutes until thickened | Remove from the fridge, top with the blueberries, and mint leaves and serve

345 KCAL | FULL OF FIBER

BAKEWELL BOSH! BALLS

Being Yorkshire lads, we wanted to give the classic Bakewell tart a twist! Add a little unflavored or vanilla protein powder to boost the protein. See photo on page 201.

MAKES 15 BALLS

1 cup rolled oats
2 tbsp almond butter
1 tbsp maple syrup
½ tsp almond extract
2 tbsp no-added-sugar
   raspberry jam
¼ cup almond flour
pinch of salt
¼ cup sliced almonds

BLENDER | AIRTIGHT CONTAINER

First, prep the ingredients | Blitz the oats in the blender until they are the texture of flour | Put the almond butter, maple syrup, almond extract, and raspberry jam in a mixing bowl and beat together to combine | Add the almond flour, ground oats, and salt and mix together until you have a thick dough | Sprinkle in a pinch of the sliced almonds and fold them into dough | Roughly chop the remaining sliced almonds

Now, roll the balls | Roll the dough into 15 equal-sized balls | Roll the balls around in the chopped sliced almonds | Put the balls in the airtight container and put the container in the fridge to chill | Consume within 3 days

63 KCAL | FULL OF FIBER

COOKIE DOUGH BOSH! BALLS

A perfect post-workout snack! Oats have slow-burn energy, health-giving beta-glucans, and fiber, and peanut butter contains healthy fats and protein. See photo on page 200.

MAKES 15 BALLS

1½ cups rolled oats
1 oz dark chocolate
1 small, ripe banana
1 tbsp crunchy peanut
   butter
2 tbsp maple syrup
½ tsp vanilla extract
1 tsp unsweetened cocoa
   powder
pinch of salt

BLENDER | AIRTIGHT CONTAINER

First, prep the ingredients | Blitz the oats in the blender until they are the texture of flour | Chop the chocolate into chips | Peel and mash the banana in a bowl with the back of a fork

Now, make the balls | Put the peanut butter, maple syrup, and vanilla extract in a bowl with the mashed banana and beat together to combine | Add the oats, cocoa powder, and salt and mix together until you have a thick dough | Sprinkle in the chocolate chips and fold them into dough | Taste and tweak to perfection

Chill the balls | Roll the dough into 15 equal-sized balls | Put the balls in the airtight container and put the container in the fridge to chill | Consume within 3 days

62 KCAL | FULL OF FIBER

BOSH! BROWNIE BALLS

Rich and delicious, these are the perfect energy boost or recovery snack after a workout. All the sweetness comes from the dates and raisins, and they are high in fiber, too. Add a teaspoon of chocolate protein powder if you want to up the protein count further. See photo on page 200.

MAKES 15 BALLS

½ cup pecans
1¼ cups rolled oats
7 oz Medjool dates
1¾ oz dark chocolate
½ tsp ground cinnamon
3½ oz flame raisins

PREHEAT OVEN TO 350°F | LINE A SHEET PAN WITH PARCHMENT PAPER | BLENDER OR FOOD PROCESSOR | AIRTIGHT CONTAINER

First, prep the pecans | Spread the pecans over the lined sheet pan, put the pan in the oven and toast for 8 minutes | Take the pecans out of the oven and let them cool down to room temperature

Now, combine the ball ingredients | Add three-quarters of the pecans to the blender or food processor with the rolled oats and blitz to a coarse meal | Pit and roughly chop the dates and add them to the blender | Roughly chop the chocolate and add two-thirds to the blender | Add the cinnamon and raisins, put the lid on, and blitz until a sticky mixture has formed | Roughly chop the remaining pecans

Now, make the balls | Transfer the mixture to a bowl | Sprinkle in the remaining pecans and chocolate and mix to combine | Make 15 equal-sized balls with the mixture (each ball should weigh about 1 oz) and put them on the pan you roasted the nuts on | Put the pan in the fridge and chill for a couple of hours | Transfer the balls to the airtight container and keep in the fridge | Eat the balls within 7 days, whenever you're in need of an energy boost

127 KCAL | FULL OF FIBER

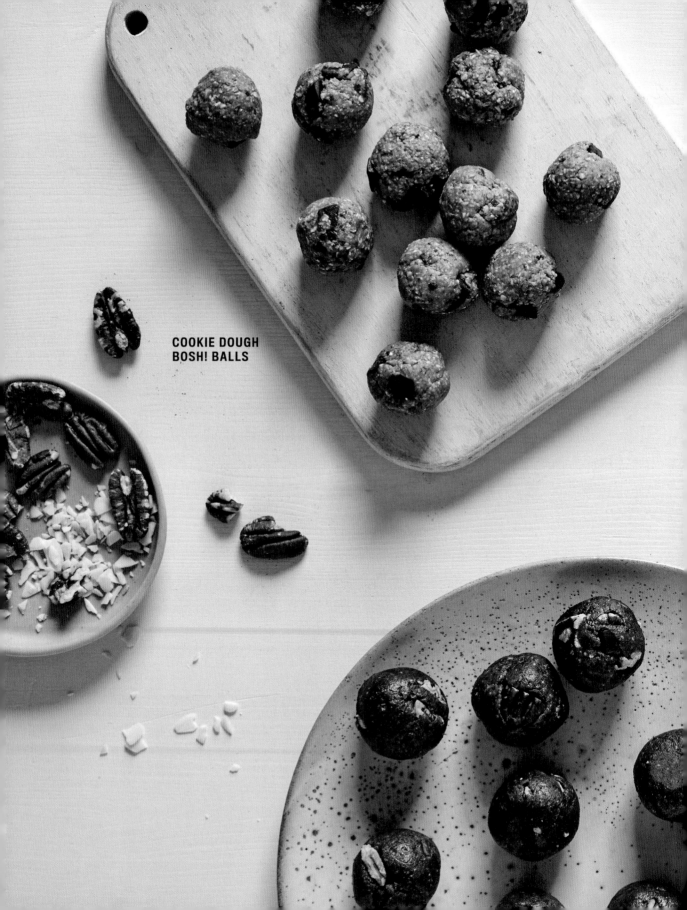

**COOKIE DOUGH
BOSH! BALLS**

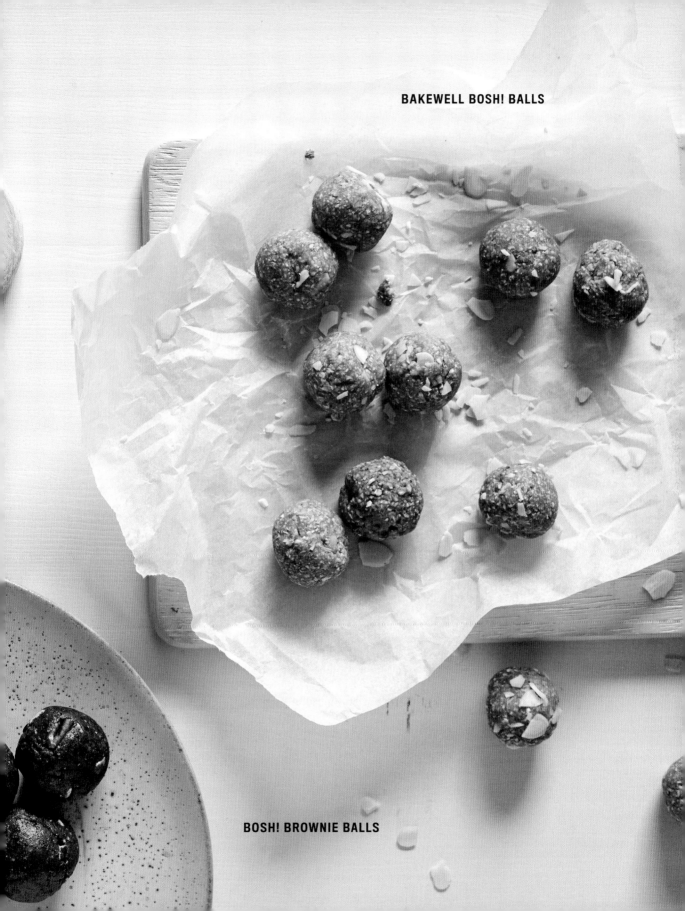

BAKEWELL BOSH! BALLS

BOSH! BROWNIE BALLS

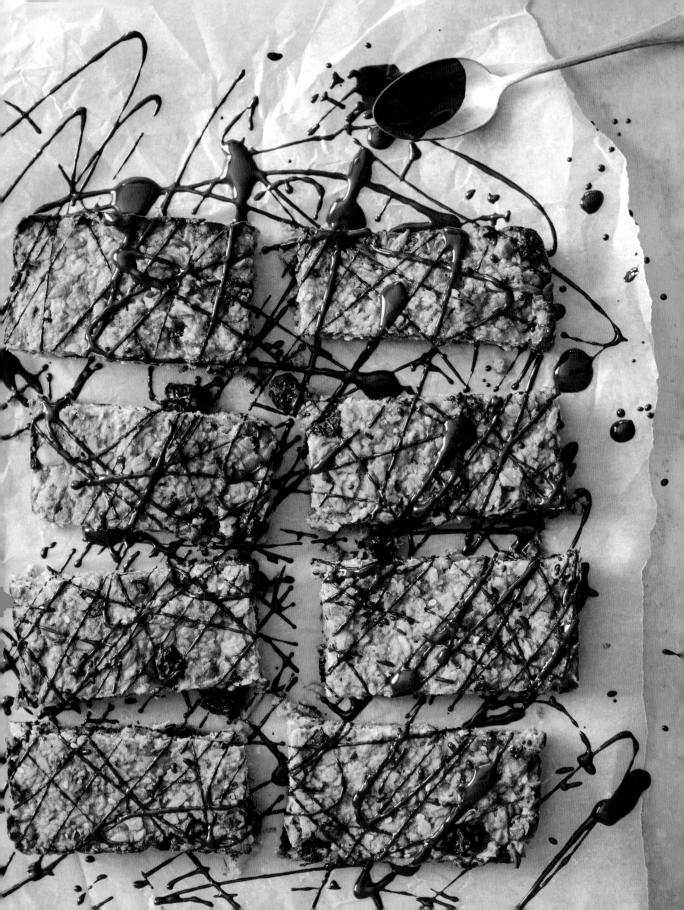

JACKED OAT BARS

The chocolatey swirls on these Jacked Oat Bars is food styling that everyone can do! They are high in fiber and goodness, coming from the banana, oats, nuts, and seeds. We've portioned them for eight, but you can chop them into sixteen if you prefer a smaller bite.

MAKES 8

- 3 ripe bananas
- 2 tbsp vegetable oil
- 2 tbsp unsweetened plant-based milk
- 2½ tbsp maple syrup
- 4½ tbsp nut butter (we use peanut)
- pinch of sea salt
- ¼ tsp ground cinnamon
- 1 oz mixed nuts
- 2½ cups rolled oats
- 1¾ oz mixed seeds (such as pumpkin, sunflower, sesame, and flaxseeds)
- 2½ oz raisins
- 1½ oz dark chocolate

PREHEAT OVEN TO 350°F | LINE AN 8-INCH BAKING PAN WITH PARCHMENT PAPER | MEDIUM SAUCEPAN

First, make the wet batter | Peel the bananas, put them in a bowl, and mash them with the back of a fork | Add the oil, milk, maple syrup, nut butter, salt, and cinnamon and mix together to form a smooth batter

Now, prep the dry ingredients | Roughly chop the mixed nuts | Add the nuts, oats, seeds, and raisins to the wet batter in the bowl and fold everything together to make a thick mixture | Transfer the mixture to the baking pan and smooth the top with the back of a spoon

Bake the oat bars | Put the pan in the oven and bake for 25–30 minutes, until golden | Remove the oat bars from the oven and let them cool down to room temperature | Remove from the pan, keeping them on the parchment paper, and cut into 8 slices

Melt the chocolate | Pour hot water into the saucepan until it's about 1¼ inches deep and bring to a boil | Reduce the heat to a simmer | Put a heatproof bowl on top of the pan, ensuring the water doesn't touch the bottom | Break the chocolate into the bowl and leave it to melt | Remove and leave to cool a little | Alternatively, melt the chocolate in a bowl in the microwave, in 15-second bursts | Drizzle the chocolate over the oat bars, leave the chocolate to set, then serve

345 KCAL | FULL OF FIBER

BANANA BERRY ICE CREAM

This super easy, silky-smooth "nice cream" combines the tartness of berries with the sweetness of banana. And it is a great way to use up bananas that are almost past their best. Experiment by stirring in some fresh berries or nuts before freezing. Or for a less sweet version, leave out the maple syrup.

MAKES ABOUT 2 PINTS (SERVES 6-8)

- 6-8 frozen ripe bananas (about 1 lb), plus extra to serve
- 10 oz frozen berries
- 3 tbsp unsweetened plant-based milk
- 1 tsp maple syrup, optional
- 1 tsp vanilla extract
- pinch of salt, optional
- fresh mint leaves, to serve

BANANAS FROZEN | BLENDER | LINE A FREEZERPROOF CONTAINER WITH PARCHMENT PAPER

First, prep the ingredients | Put the frozen bananas and berries, milk, maple syrup (if using), and vanilla extract in the blender and blitz into a thick, smooth cream (use a tamper to force the berries into the blender if you need to) | Taste and tweak to perfection—you want to get the perfect level of sweetness (add a touch of salt if you like)

Time to freeze the mixture | Put the mixture in the lined container and smooth the top with a spatula | Put the box in the freezer and freeze for a few hours until frozen through | Remove from the freezer about 30 minutes before serving, so it has a chance to soften | Serve with extra frozen berries and a garnish of mint leaves

145 KCAL | LOW FAT | FULL OF FIBER

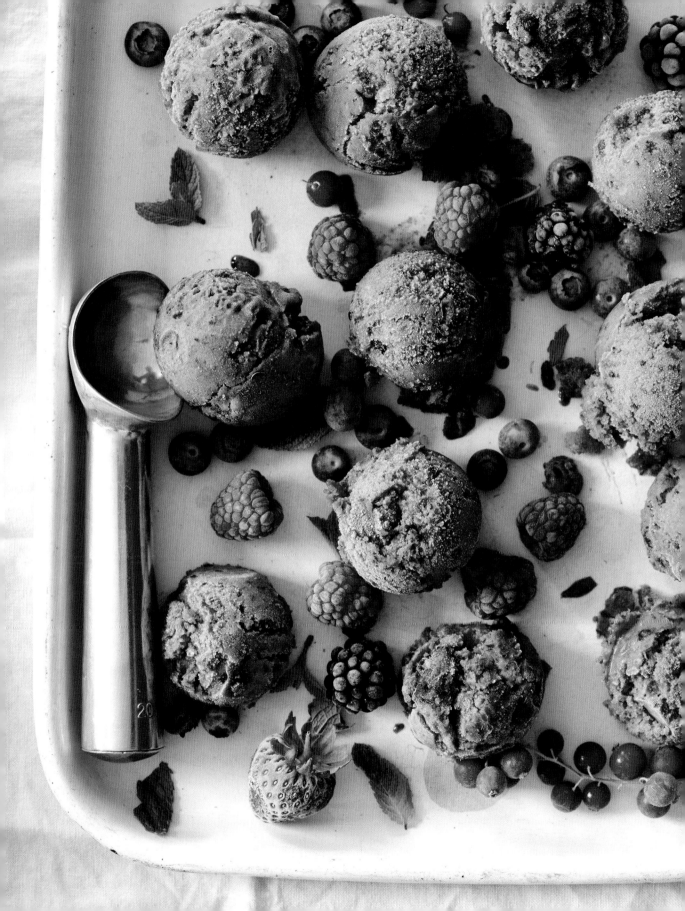

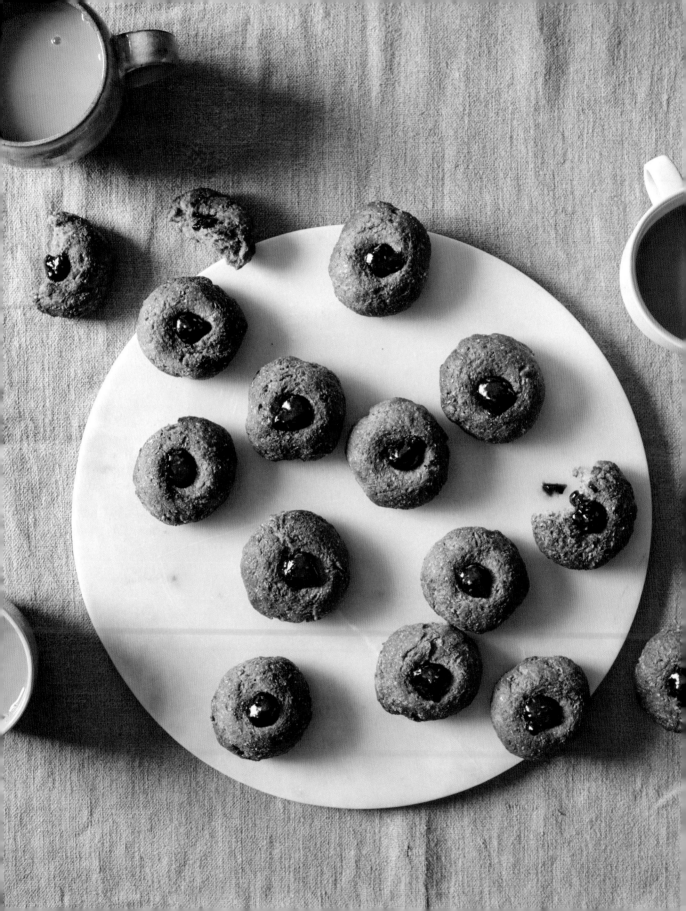

PB&J THUMBPRINT COOKIES

Could these be the simplest, easiest cookies to make, ever? Maybe. Are they delicious? Definitely! We simply mix flour, nut butter, and bananas together, along with good old PB&J flavors. The thumbprint helps them cook more quickly—and they're fun to do! Try making them with the kids.

MAKES 12 COOKIES

2 small ripe bananas

scant ⅓ cup nut butter (we use almond)

heaping ¾ cup whole wheat flour

6 tbsp no-added-sugar jam (we use raspberry)

¾ tsp baking powder

pinch of salt

First, make the cookie dough | Peel the bananas, put them in a mixing bowl, and mash with the back of a fork | Add the nut butter, flour, 4 tbsp of the jam, the baking powder, and salt to the bowl and stir well to combine | Knead the dough with your hand to bring it together if necessary

Now, make and bake the cookies | Divide the dough into 12 equal-sized pieces | Roll each piece into a ball then flatten into cookie shapes 1½–2 inches in diameter, pushing your thumb into the top of each cookie—this acts as a well for the jam after the first round of baking | Put the cookies on the lined baking sheet, put the pan in the oven and bake for 10 minutes | Take the pan out of the oven and spoon equal amounts of the remaining jam into the thumbprint wells on the top of the cookies | Put the pan back in the oven and bake for another 5–10 minutes until the dough is golden brown | Remove the pan from the oven, transfer the cookies to the cooling rack, and leave to cool to room temperature before eating

149 KCAL | FULL OF FIBER

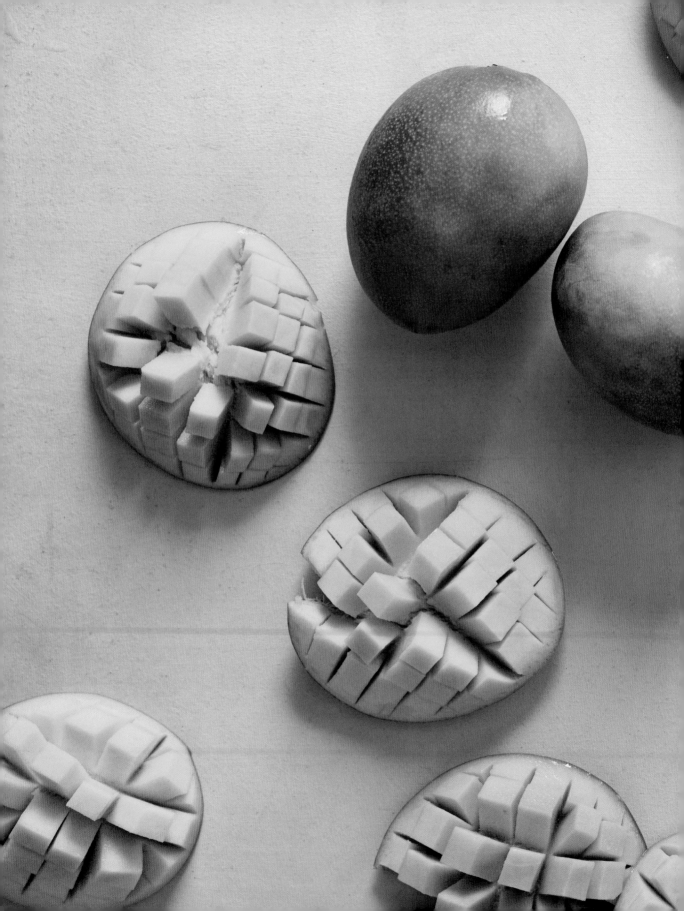

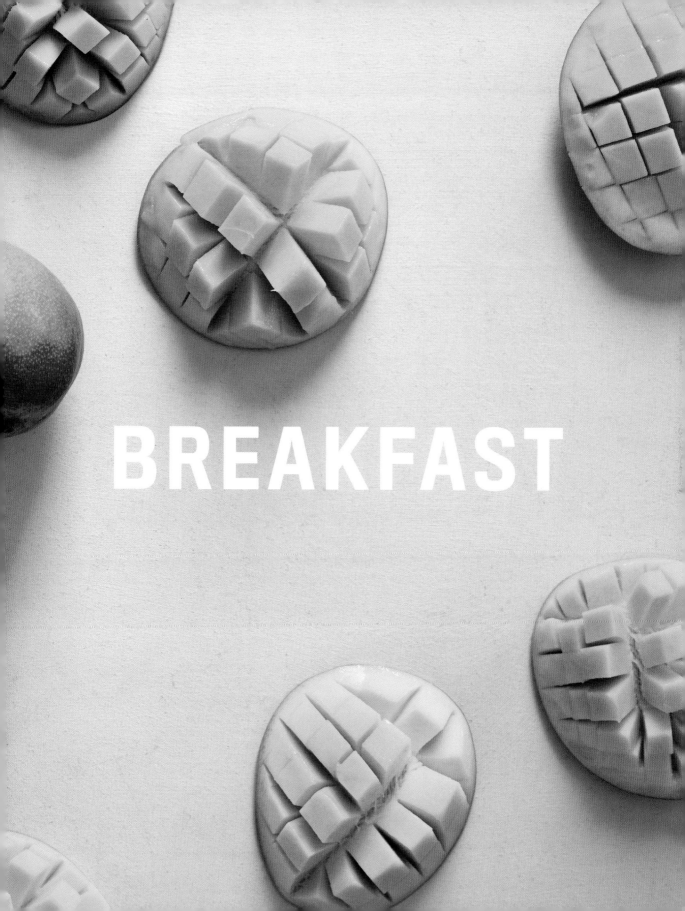

BREAKFAST

GREEN GODDESS SMOOTHIE

SERVES 2 (MAKES ABOUT 2 CUPS)

1 apple
1 banana
2 oz fresh spinach leaves
1 oz kale
1 cup oat milk
1 tsp maple syrup
2 tsp ground flaxseed, optional
scant ¼ cup unflavored or vanilla vegan protein powder, optional

We like to drink this smoothie most mornings, to get a power-packed nutrient-rich start to the day. Try batching the smoothie ingredients and keeping individual servings in freezer bags for quick preparation. We usually make it with oat milk that has been fortified with calcium and vitamin D. See photo on page 212.

POWER BLENDER

Core the apple, peel the banana, and cut them into chunks | Put the spinach and kale in the blender with a splash of the oat milk and blend | Add the fruit, the rest of the oat milk, the maple syrup, flaxseed, and protein powder, if using, put the lid on, and blend until completely smooth | Pour into glasses and serve immediately

229 KCAL | LOW FAT | FULL OF FIBER | PROTEIN PACKED

BERRY BOOST SMOOTHIE

SERVES 2 (MAKES ABOUT 2 CUPS)

10 oz frozen berries
⅔ cup rolled oats
scant ¼ cup unflavored or vanilla vegan protein powder, optional
2 tsp ground flaxseed, optional
1 tsp maple syrup, optional
1¼ cups unsweetened plant-based milk

This smoothie is low in fat and full of antioxidants, and if you use the protein powder, it's packed with protein. Using frozen berries means it's easy to make, even in winter when berries aren't in season. To make this more substantial, try serving with some fresh fruit to make a smoothie bowl. See photo on page 213.

POWER BLENDER

Put all the ingredients in the blender | Put the lid on and blend until very smooth (loosen with a little water or extra milk if needed) | Pour into glasses and serve immediately

298 KCAL | LOW FAT | FULL OF FIBER | PROTEIN PACKED

BANANA, OAT & NUT SMOOTHIE

This gorgeous smoothie is the perfect thing to help you recover from a workout. We like to add protein powder and flaxseeds to give us a powerful kick-start to our day. Go for milks that are fortified with calcium and vitamin D. See photo on page 213.

SERVES 2 (MAKES ABOUT 2½ CUPS)

2 small bananas

⅔ cup rolled oats

scant ¼ cup unflavored banana or vanilla vegan protein powder, optional

2 tbsp smooth nut butter

2 tsp ground flaxseed, optional

1 tsp vanilla extract

small pinch of salt

2 cups unsweetened plant-based milk

1 tsp maple syrup, optional

POWER BLENDER

Peel the bananas and put them in the blender with all the remaining ingredients | Put the lid on and blend until smooth (loosen with a little water if needed) | Pour into glasses and serve immediately

459 KCAL | FULL OF FIBER | PROTEIN PACKED

GREEN GODDESS SMOOTHIE

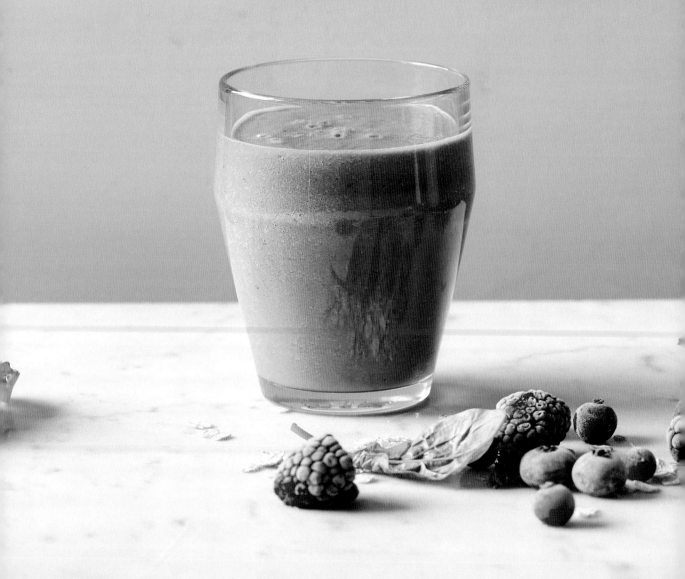

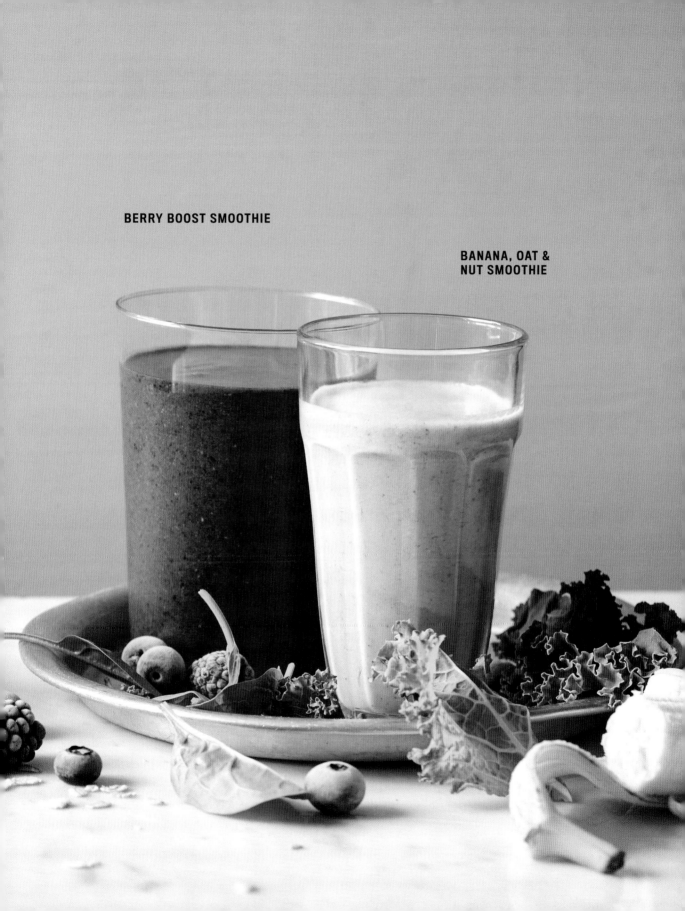

BERRY BOOST SMOOTHIE

**BANANA, OAT &
NUT SMOOTHIE**

CHARLIE'S SAUSAGE SCRAMBLE

Charlie is our trusty videographer, occasionally the hands in our videos, and always a firm advocate for scrambled tofu. Fluffy and light yet filling, this dish is a wonderful way to start the day. It's absolutely jam-packed with protein, too, containing all nine of the essential amino acids the body requires.

SERVES 2 FOR A BIG BRUNCH

- 7 oz firm tofu
- 2 vegan sausages
- 7 oz silken tofu
- 1 garlic clove
- 2 scallions
- 2 oz fresh spinach leaves
- ½ tbsp olive oil
- ¼ tsp ground turmeric
- pinch of black salt, optional
- ½ tsp soy sauce
- salt and black pepper
- 4 slices whole wheat sourdough bread, to serve

PREHEAT OVEN TO 350°F | TOFU PRESS OR 2 CLEAN TEA TOWELS AND A WEIGHT SUCH AS A HEAVY BOOK | SHEET PAN | BLENDER | FINE GRATER OR MICROPLANE | SKILLET

Press the firm tofu using a tofu press or place it between two clean tea towels, lay it on a plate, and put a weight on top | Leave for a few minutes to drain off any liquid and firm up

Put the sausages on the sheet pan and cook in the oven for 20 minutes

Blitz the silken tofu in the blender until smooth | Peel and grate the garlic | Trim and thinly slice the scallions | Wash, dry, and roughly chop the spinach | Crumble the pressed tofu into small pieces

Heat the olive oil in the skillet over medium heat | Add some of the scallions (saving a tablespoon of the green parts for garnish) and cook, stirring, for 30 seconds | Add the garlic and stir for another 30 seconds | Reduce the heat, add the turmeric, black salt (if using), and soy sauce and stir to combine | Take the pan off the heat

Take the sausages out of the oven and carefully cut them into ⅓-inch chunks | Return the pan to medium heat, add the sausage pieces, and cook for 2–3 minutes, stirring, until the sausage starts to crisp up | Reduce the heat, add the blended silken tofu, and stir until the silken tofu has taken on the color of the turmeric and started to bubble | Crumble the firm tofu into the pan and fold it with the other ingredients for 2 minutes until it's completely warmed through | Add the spinach and fold it into the sausage scramble | Taste and season to perfection with salt and pepper

Toast the bread | Serve the scramble on the toast and garnish with the remaining scallion

271 KCAL | LOW SUGAR | FULL OF FIBER | PROTEIN PACKED

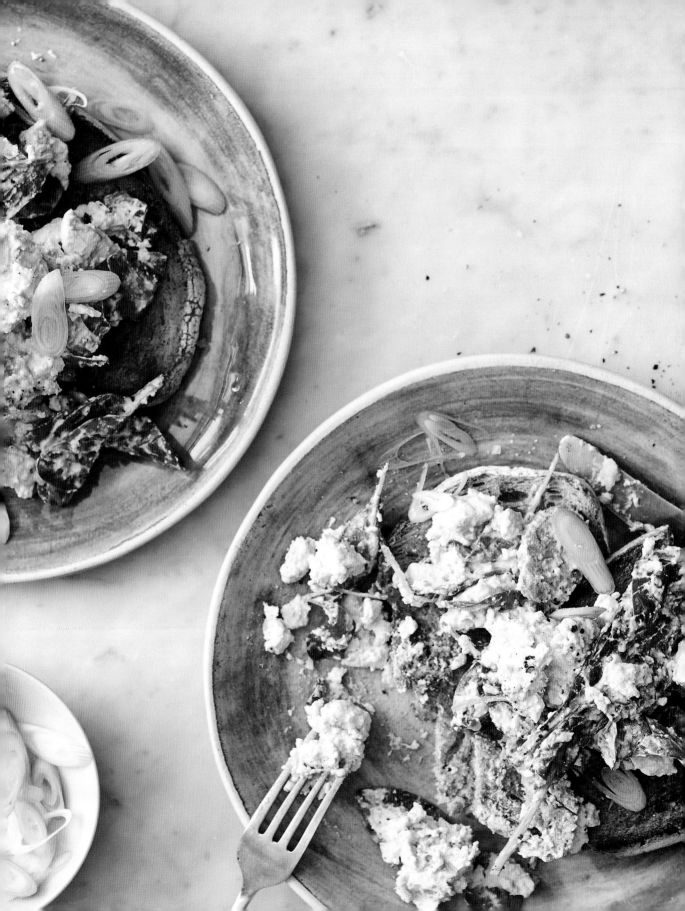

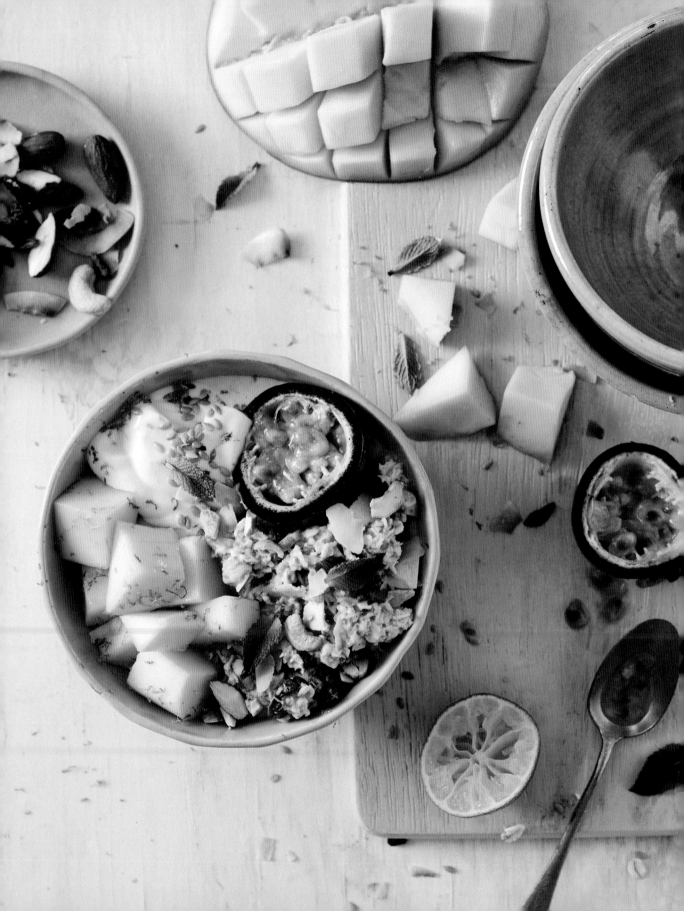

TROPICAL OVERNIGHT OATS

Make these overnight oats in advance and simply grab-and-go in the morning. This tropical combination brings a delicious taste of sunshine to start the day, and there is no added sugar, letting the sweetness of the fruits shine through. Mango is full of vitamin C and the oats are packed with beta-glucans (which are great for your heart), as well as releasing energy slowly.

SERVES 2

1¼ cups rolled oats
1 tbsp almonds (skin on)
1 tbsp cashews
1tbsp flaked coconut
¾ oz dried fruit
1 cup unsweetened plant-based milk
pinch of salt
1 medium mango
1 lime
¾ cup unsweetened plant-based yogurt
small handful of fresh mint leaves
½ tbsp flaxseeds
1 passionfruit

THE NIGHT BEFORE | PREHEAT OVEN TO 350°F | SHEET PAN | FINE GRATER OR MICROPLANE | 3 AIRTIGHT CONTAINERS

The night before you want to eat your tropical overnight oats | Place the oats, almonds, cashews, and flaked coconut on the sheet pan (keeping them separate) and bake in the oven for 5 minutes, until golden brown (be careful they don't burn)

Place the oats and dried fruit in an airtight container, pour in the milk, and add the salt | Stir everything together, put the lid on, and put the container in the fridge

Roughly chop the toasted nuts and put them in a separate container along with the flaked coconut | Put the lid on and set to one side

Slice the mango lengthwise down either side of the pit, spoon out the flesh, cut the mango into bite-sized chunks, and put the chunks in a container | Zest the lime into the container | Put the lid on the container and put the container in the fridge

The following morning | Layer the overnight oats, nuts, chopped fruit, yogurt, mint leaves, and flaxseeds | Halve the passionfruit | Serve the oats immediately, with the passionfruit halves

491 KCAL | FULL OF FIBER | PROTEIN PACKED

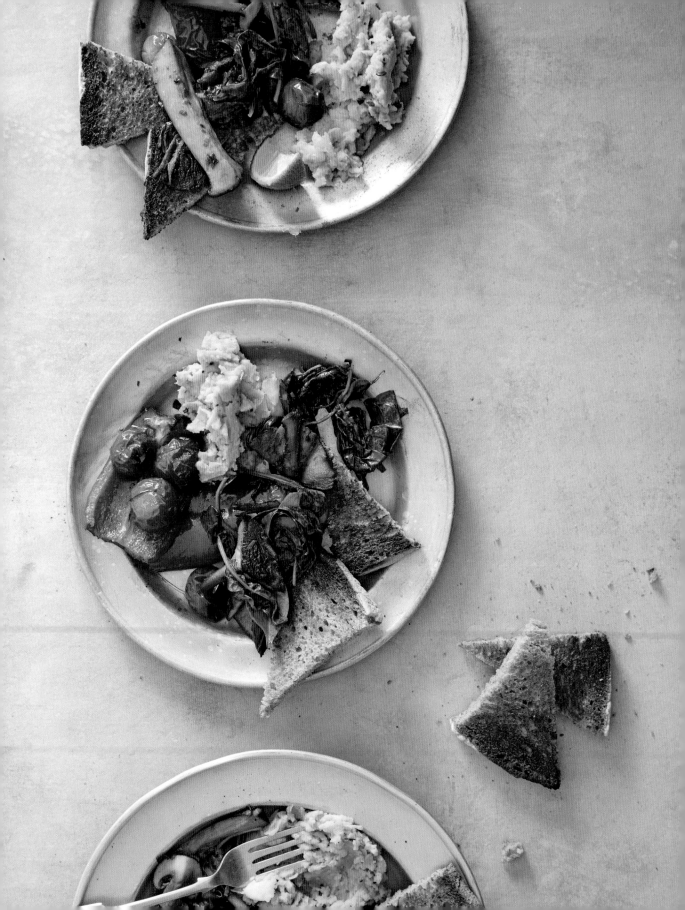

MEXI BREAKFAST

There are so many surprising textures and punchy flavors on this plate, it's the perfect way to kick off your Saturday! The fresh avocado is a great source of unsaturated fat, and tomatoes are packed with lycopene, which is great for immunity. It's one of our favorite eat-the-rainbow dishes.

SERVES 4

8 slices whole wheat bread
½ cup fresh cilantro leaves
salt and black pepper

FOR THE SMOKY ROASTED RED PEPPERS

2 red bell peppers
7 oz cherry tomatoes
½ tbsp olive oil
1 tsp smoked paprika

FOR THE CREAMY, PROTEIN-PACKED AVOCADO SMASH

1 (14 oz) can butter beans or lima beans
1 ripe avocado
1 lime
chile flakes, to taste

FOR THE SPICY MIXED MUSHROOMS & GREENS

1 large shallot
1 large garlic clove
14 oz mixed mushrooms
½ tbsp olive oil
1–2 tsp cayenne pepper
1 lime
10 oz baby spinach

PREHEAT OVEN TO 400°F | LINE A SHEET PAN | POTATO MASHER | FINE GRATER OR MICROPLANE | SKILLET

Start by making the smoky roasted red peppers | Trim, core, and quarter the peppers and put them in a bowl | Add the cherry tomatoes, olive oil, and smoked paprika, season with salt and pepper, and toss to coat | Tip the vegetables onto the lined sheet pan, put the pan in the oven and roast for 20–25 minutes

To make the avocado smash, first drain, rinse, and mash the butter beans in a bowl with the potato masher | Halve and carefully pit the avocado by tapping the pit firmly with the heel of a knife so that it lodges in the pit, then twist and remove | Scoop the avocado flesh into the bowl of butter beans | Halve the lime and squeeze in the juice | Mash everything together, taste and season to perfection with salt, pepper, and chile flakes

Now, make the spicy mushrooms and greens | Peel and finely dice the shallot | Peel and grate the garlic | Roughly chop the mushrooms | Heat the oil in the skillet over medium heat | Add the shallot and a pinch of salt and stir for 2 minutes | Add the garlic and stir for 30 seconds | Increase the heat to medium-high and add the mushrooms and cayenne pepper | Cook for 8–10 minutes, stirring occasionally, until the mushrooms are completely cooked | Halve the lime and squeeze the juice over the mushrooms | Add the spinach and stir the leaves into the mushrooms for 1–2 minutes, until well wilted | Season with more salt and some pepper

Now you're ready to plate up your breakfast | Toast the bread and cut the slices into triangles to make toast "tortilla chips" | Serve the chips with your roasted red peppers, avocado smash, and mixed mushrooms and greens | Garnish with the cilantro and serve immediately

565 KCAL | LOW FAT | LOW SUGAR | FULL OF FIBER | PROTEIN PACKED

MAPLE PECAN GRANOLA

Oats are a great source of fiber and slow-release energy. Nuts and seeds will help make sure you're getting enough healthy fats in your diet. We do add sugar to our granola as it helps it clump together as it cooks, but you can leave it out if you don't mind it being more flaky. Try some in the Summer Berry Granola Bowl on page 229?

MAKES 8 SERVINGS

2 tbsp vegetable oil
1/2 cup maple syrup
1 tsp ground cinnamon
1 tsp vanilla extract
pinch of salt
4⅓ cup rolled oats
½ cup pecans
1¾ oz mixed seeds (such as pumpkin, sunflower, sesame, and flaxseeds)
¼ sliced almonds
⅓ cup flame raisins
⅓ cup dried cranberries

First, prep the wet ingredients | Mix the vegetable oil, maple syrup, cinnamon, vanilla extract, and salt in a large bowl

Now, prep the dry ingredients | Put 1¼ cups of the oats in a blender or food processor and blitz until coarsely ground | Roughly chop the pecans | Add the blitzed oats, whole oats, mixed seeds, sliced almonds, and chopped pecans to the bowl of wet ingredients and use your hands to press and combine | Tip the mixture out onto the lined sheet pan and firmly press the mixture down with your hands to create a solid layer

Now, bake the granola | Put the pan in the oven and bake for 10 minutes | Remove the pan from the oven and loosely mix the granola around with a spoon | Put the pan back in the oven and bake for another 15 minutes

Cool the granola and store until you're ready to eat | Take the pan out of the oven and let the granola cool to room temperature | Stir the raisins and cranberries into the granola, and transfer the granola to the airtight jar | Consume within 10 days

295 KCAL | FULL OF FIBER

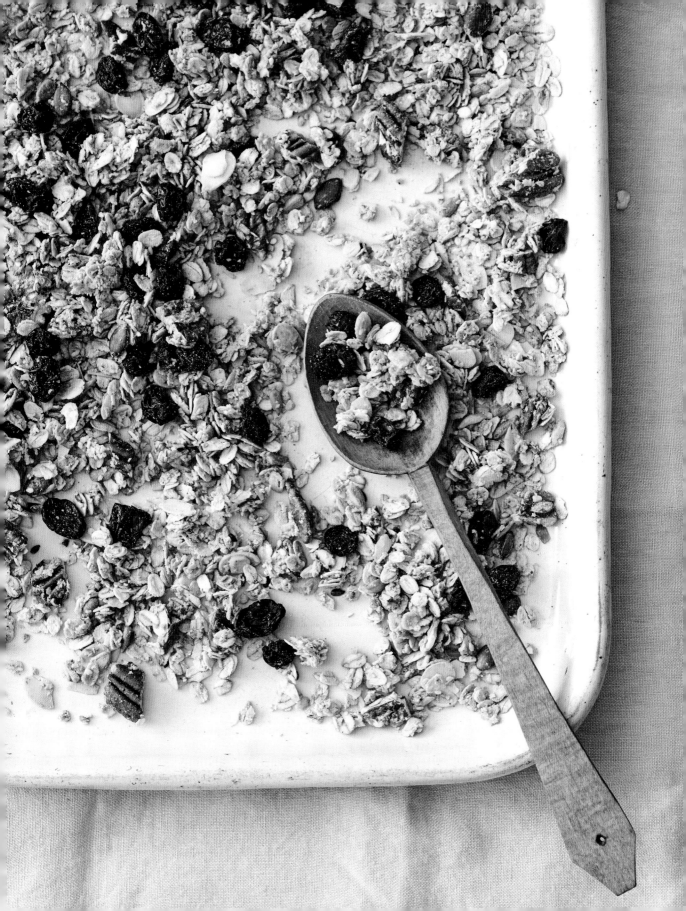

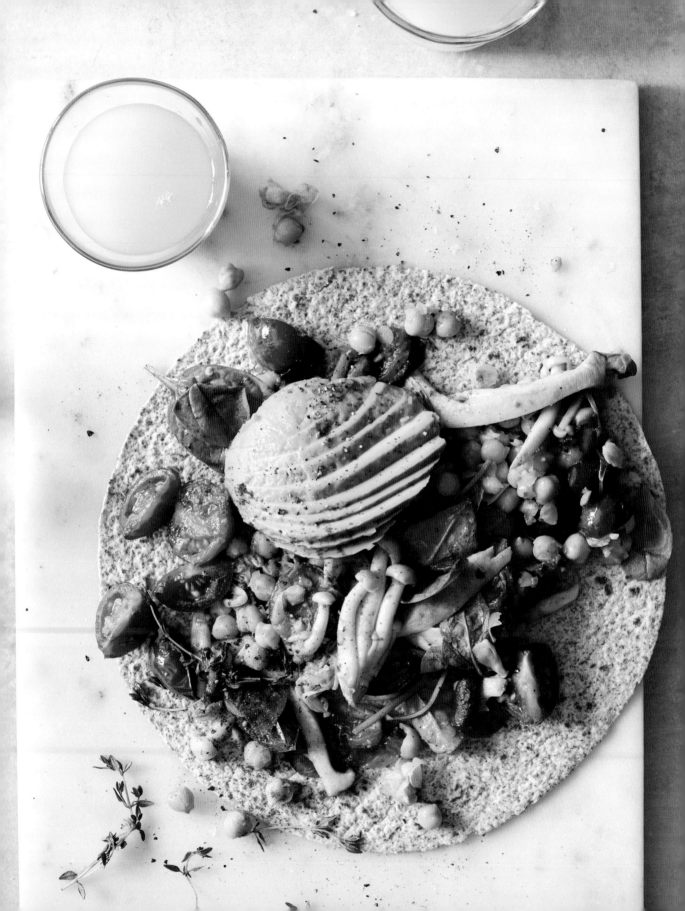

BARCELONA BREAKFAST BURRITO

This recipe combines all our favorite elements of a fried breakfast in a handy wrap. It has some delicious tapas-like flavors going on, courtesy of the thyme, smoked paprika, garlic, and lemon. Go for whole wheat tortillas for higher fiber.

SERVES 2

1 garlic clove
1 shallot
7 oz mixed mushrooms
5 oz cherry tomatoes
1 (14 oz) can chickpeas
½ oz fresh thyme sprigs
3½ oz baby spinach
1 small ripe avocado (about 2.5 oz)
2 tsp olive oil
½ tsp smoked paprika
½ tbsp soy sauce
½ lemon
2 large whole wheat tortillas
salt and black pepper

FINE GRATER OR MICROPLANE | POTATO MASHER | MEDIUM SKILLET

First, prep your ingredients | Peel and grate the garlic | Peel and finely chop the shallot | Clean the mushrooms and cut them into bite-sized chunks | Roughly chop the cherry tomatoes | Drain and rinse the chickpeas, place in a bowl, and lightly squish with the potato masher or a fork | Pick the thyme leaves from the sprigs and roughly chop | Wash, dry, and roughly chop the spinach | Halve and carefully pit the avocado by tapping the pit firmly with the heel of a knife so that it lodges in the pit, then twist and remove | Scoop out and slice the avocado flesh

Now, cook the filling | Heat the oil in the skillet over medium-low heat | Add the shallot and a small pinch of salt and stir for 30 seconds | Add the garlic and stir for another minute | Add the mushrooms, half the tomatoes, and the thyme and cook for another 2–3 minutes

Add the mashed chickpeas, smoked paprika, and soy sauce and sauté for another 5–6 minutes, folding everything together regularly with a wooden spoon | Squeeze the juice of the half lemon over the mixture, sprinkle over the remaining tomatoes, and fold the mixture to combine | Season to taste with salt and pepper | Remove from the heat and fold in the spinach | Spoon the mixture into the middle of the tortillas, place the avocado slices on top, and serve immediately, wrapping the burritos at the breakfast table

BOSH! BARS

We've all been there: grabbing something unhealthy to quickly satisfy an urge or craving. Making these crunchy, fruity bars will ensure you'll always have something nutritious and delicious to nibble on! These may not be low in sugar, but all their sweetness comes from natural fruity goodness. High in fiber, they will keep you feeling full for longer.

MAKES 10 BARS

- 1¾ cups rolled oats
- 1¾ oz mixed nuts (such as almonds, hazelnuts, walnuts, cashews)
- 3 tbsp unsweetened shredded coconut
- 1¾ mixed seeds (such as pumpkin, sunflower, sesame, and flaxseed)
- 3½ oz mixed dried fruit (such as currants, golden raisins, dried cherries, apricots)
- 3½ oz Medjool dates
- 1 orange
- 2 tbsp ground flaxseed
- 1½ tsp ground cinnamon
- pinch of salt
- 2 small bananas (about 5 oz)
- 1 tbsp vanilla extract
- ¼ cup almond butter

PREHEAT OVEN TO 350°F | LINE AN 8-INCH SQUARE BAKING PAN | 2 SHEET PANS | FINE GRATER OR MICROPLANE | COOLING RACK | AIRTIGHT CONTAINER

Put the oats, nuts, coconut, and seeds on the 2 sheet pans, keeping them roughly separated | Put the pans in the oven and toast for 5–7 minutes

Roughly chop the dried fruit and pit and chop the dates and put them in a bowl | Zest and juice the orange into the bowl and allow the fruit to soak for 5 minutes | Remove the toasted ingredients from the oven and set aside to cool | Roughly chop the nuts | Add all the toasted ingredients to the bowl of fruit | Add the ground flaxseed, cinnamon, and salt and fold to combine

Peel the bananas, put them in a mixing bowl, and mash to a smooth paste | Stir the vanilla and almond butter into the banana to combine | Tip the oat and fruit mixture into the wet ingredients and stir to combine

Tip the mixture into the baking pan | Spread it out with a spatula, making sure the mixture is smooth on top | Put the pan in the oven and bake for 20–25 minutes, until the mixture is beginning to turn golden | Take the pan out of the oven, place it on a cooling rack, and allow to cool completely | Remove from the pan, cut into 10 bars, and transfer to an airtight container

242 KCAL | FULL OF FIBER

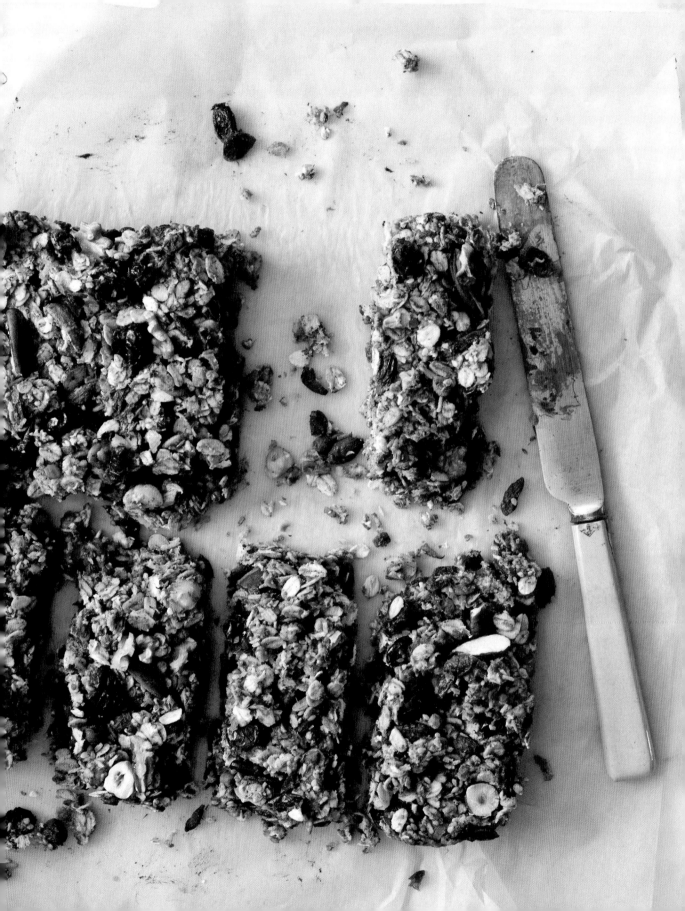

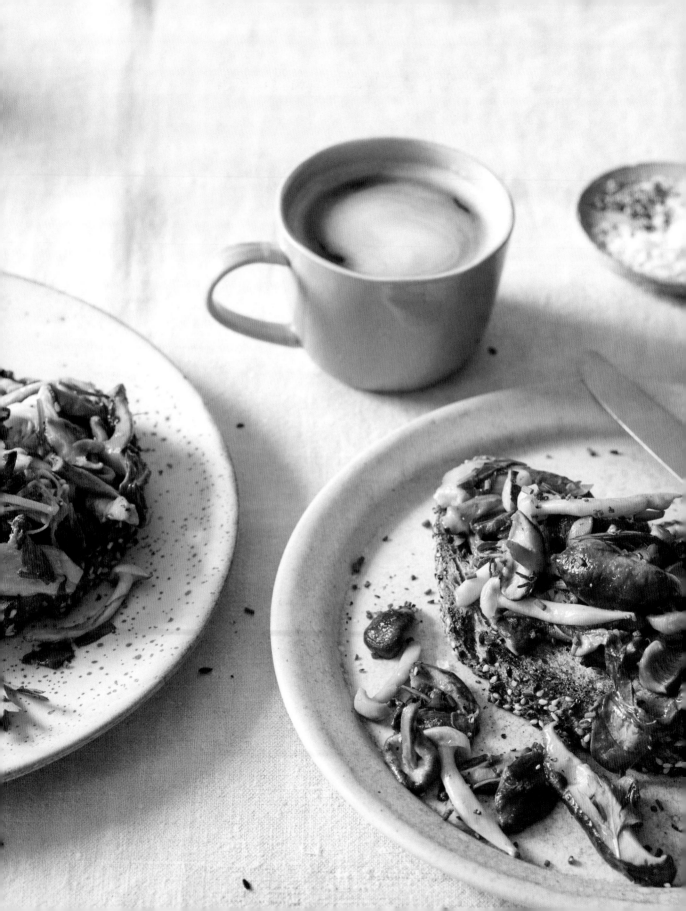

BREAKFAST OF CHAMPIGNONS

Sometimes keeping things simple is the key to satisfaction. This makes quite a large serving of the mushrooms, so you can serve it with more toast if you like. Mushrooms are a rich source of lots of vitamins and minerals, including vitamin B5 and selenium. They are also a source of potassium and vitamin D.

SERVES 2

14 oz mushrooms
   of choice
2 tsp olive oil
2 garlic cloves
6 sprigs fresh thyme
scant ½ cup fresh parsley
   leaves
3 chives
2 slices whole wheat
   seeded bread
7 oz baby spinach
salt and black pepper

MEDIUM SKILLET | FINE GRATER OR MICROPLANE

Roughly chop the mushrooms into bite-sized pieces

Heat the olive oil in the skillet over medium-high heat | Add the mushrooms with a pinch of salt and cook, stirring, for 8–10 minutes

Meanwhile, peel and grate the garlic | Pick the thyme leaves and roughly chop | Finely chop the parsley and chives | Add the garlic and thyme to the pan and cook, stirring, for 2 minutes (add more oil if the pan dries out, to prevent the mushrooms catching and burning)

Toast the bread | Remove the pan from the heat, add the spinach, and stir until wilted

Plate up | Place the mushroom mixture on top of the toast, sprinkle with parsley and chives, season with salt and pepper, and serve immediately

277 KCAL | LOW FAT | LOW SUGAR | FULL OF FIBER | PROTEIN PACKED

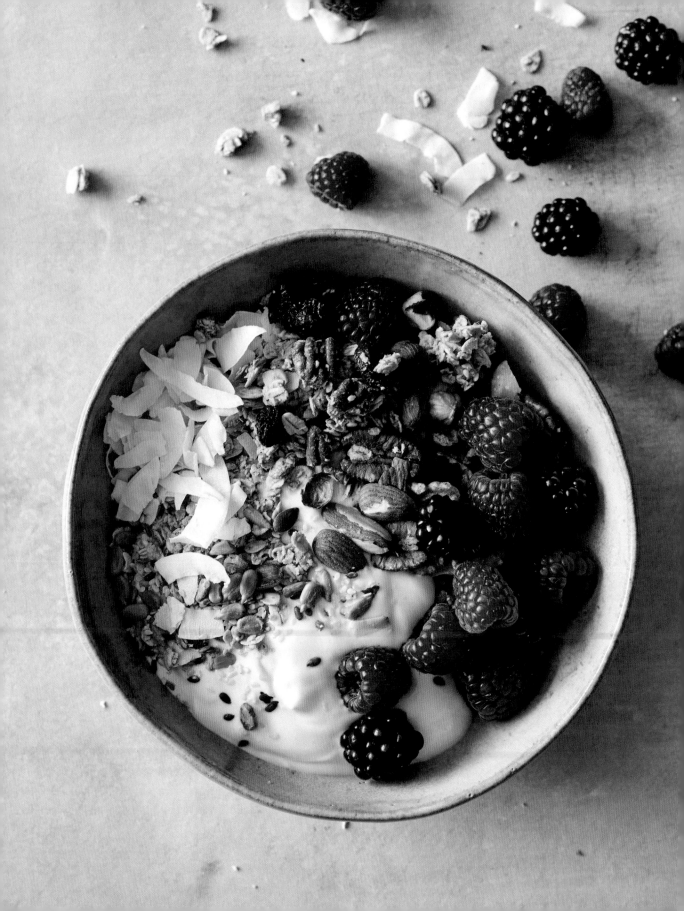

SUMMER BERRY GRANOLA BOWL

What better way to start the day than with a handful of berries, some granola, nuts, seeds, and coconut flakes? This bowl is incredibly quick to put together and is full of natural sweetness and satisfying crunch. In addition to all the antioxidants and goodness in the berries, the yogurt is probiotic, which supports good gut health. Go for yogurt fortified with calcium and vitamin D.

SERVES 1

1 oz mixed nuts

½ cup unsweetened plant-based yogurt

1½ oz plant-baseds granola (store-bought or see our recipe on page 220)

⅓ cup fresh blackberries

heaping ⅓ cup fresh raspberries

1 tsp mixed seeds (such as pumpkin, sesame, or flaxseeds)

1 tbsp flaked coconut

PREHEAT OVEN TO 350°F | SHEET PAN

Spread the nuts out on the sheet pan | Put the pan in the oven and roast for 6–7 minutes, until the nuts are lightly toasted | Remove the pan from the oven, transfer to a cutting board, and roughly chop

Put the yogurt in a bowl | Add the granola, chopped nuts, berries, seeds, and flaked coconut and serve immediately

484 KCAL | LOW SUGAR | FULL OF FIBER | PROTEIN PACKED

HEALTHY BANANA
FRENCH TOAST

Have you ever heard of French toast that was low in fat and sat fat? Well, we've done it! Delicious and moreish, but also fairly healthy, this weekend breakfast is a source of protein, too. For extra flavor try toasting the coconut flakes in the oven.

SERVES 2

FOR THE FRENCH TOAST

1 ripe banana
1 cup unsweetened almond milk
½ tsp vanilla extract
¼ tsp ground nutmeg
½ tsp ground cinnamon
1½ tsp all-purpose flour
pinch of sea salt
1 tsp maple syrup
4 slices whole wheat bread

FOR THE BERRY SYRUP

14 oz mixed frozen berries
¼ cup water
1 tbsp maple syrup

TO SERVE

1 small, ripe banana
¼ cup plant-based yogurt
10–12 fresh berries
1 tbsp flaked coconut

First, make the French toast | Peel and mash the banana with the back of a fork in a wide, shallow bowl | Add the milk, vanilla extract, nutmeg, cinnamon, flour, salt, and maple syrup and mix well to combine | Lay the bread slices in the mixture for 15 seconds or so, turning it so it soaks through, then lay them on the lined sheet pan | Put the pan in the oven and bake the French toast for 30 minutes, until golden, turning the slices halfway through

Now, make the berry syrup | Put the small saucepan over medium heat | Add the berries, water, and maple syrup and simmer for 15–20 minutes, until the liquid has reduced, stirring regularly | Halfway through cooking, gently mash the fruit with the back of a spoon

Time to serve | Peel and slice the remaining banana | Plate up the toast, top with the berry syrup, the banana slices, yogurt, fresh berries, and coconut, and serve

536 KCAL | LOW FAT | FULL OF FIBER | PROTEIN PACKED

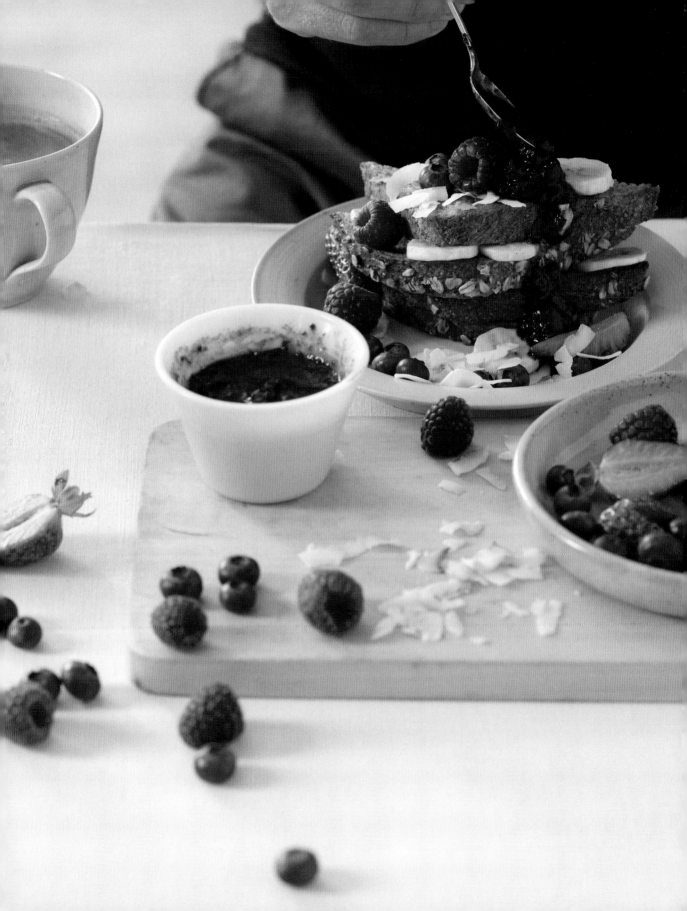

GARDEN PARTY BREAKFAST BOWL

This is a fun take on a healthy breakfast. It's like a breakfast salad, packed with fresh and vibrant flavors and textures. To up the protein content, you could add a teaspoon of vegan vanilla protein powder to the yogurt first.

SERVES 4

⅓ cup almonds (skin on)

1 small watermelon (about 1 lb 5 oz)

10 oz strawberries

1 lime

1 sprig fresh mint

½ cucumber

1 tbsp maple syrup

7 oz blueberries

½ cup unsweetened plant-based yogurt

1 tbsp mixed seeds (such as pumpkin, sunflower, sesame, and flaxseed)

PREHEAT OVEN TO 350°F | SHEET PAN | BLENDER | SALAD BOWL

First, prep your ingredients | Put the almonds on the sheet pan, put the pan in the oven, and roast for 8–10 minutes, until fragrant | Peel the watermelon and cut the flesh into bite-sized chunks | Hull and halve or quarter the strawberries | Halve the lime | Pick and thinly slice the mint leaves or keep them whole if they are small | Halve the cucumber lengthwise and scrape the watery seeds into the blender with a spoon | Cut the cucumber into bite-sized chunks or slices and place in the salad bowl | Squeeze half of the lime juice into the blender (cut the other half into quarters) | Add the maple syrup to the blender and blitz into a smooth dressing | Take the almonds out of the oven and roughly chop them

Now, build the salad | Add the watermelon to the salad bowl | Drizzle over the dressing and toss to coat | Add the strawberries and blueberries to the bowl and gently toss to combine | Divide among four bowls | Spoon over the yogurt | Sprinkle over the mint, almonds, and seeds and serve immediately, with the remaining lime quarters

255 KCAL | LOW FAT | FULL OF FIBER | PROTEIN PACKED

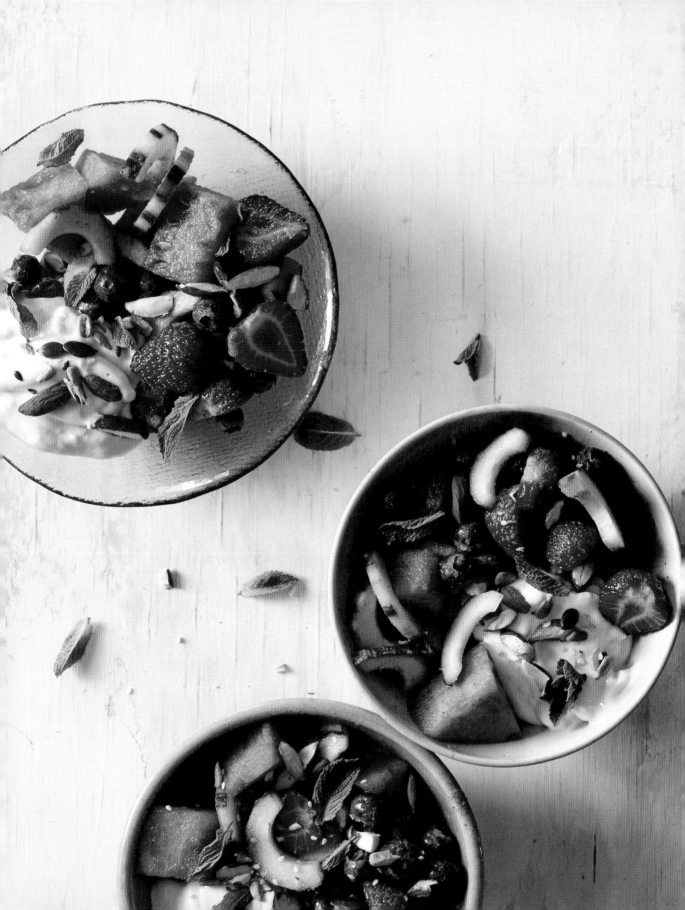

INDEX

START YOUR OWN PERSONALIZED MEAL PLAN AT WWW.BOSH.TV